DIFFICULT DIAGNOSES IN ADULT COMMUNICATION DISORDERS

DIFFICULT DIAGNOSES IN ADULT COMMUNICATION DISORDERS

EDITED BY

NANCY HELM-ESTABROOKS, Sc.D.
BOSTON VA MEDICAL CENTER
BOSTON UNIVERSITY SCHOOL OF MEDICINE
BOSTON, MASSACHUSETTS

JAMES L. ATEN, PH.D.
LONG BEACH VA MEDICAL CENTER
LONG BEACH, CALIFORNIA

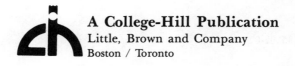

A College-Hill Publication
Little, Brown and Company
Boston / Toronto

College-Hill Press
A Division of
Little, Brown and Company (Inc.)
34 Beacon Street
Boston, Massachusetts 02108

Library of Congress Cataloging in Publication Data
Main entry under title:

Difficult diagnoses in adult communication disorders / edited by Nancy
    Helm-Estabrooks, James Aten.
        p.   cm.
    Bibliography.
    Includes index.
    1. Communicative disorders — Case studies.   I. Helm-Estabrooks,
    Nancy, 1940–   II. Aten, James, 1931–
    RC423.D54   1989   88-23741
    616.85′5–dc19   CIP

ISBN 0-316-35507-0

Printed in the United States of America

CONTENTS

SECTION I
QUESTION OF NEUROGENIC ETIOLOGY IN ADULTS
WITH ACQUIRED FLUENCY DISORDERS

SECTION II
UNUSUAL BEHAVIORS ASSOCIATED WITH HEAD INJURY

SECTION VI
DIAGNOSTIC AND MANAGEMENT STRATEGIES FOR DYSTONIC AND DYSARTHRIC PATIENTS

SECTION VII
DIAGNOSING DEMENTIA IN PATIENTS WITH EARLY ONSET OF SPEECH–LANGUAGE PROBLEMS

PREFACE

*A*t the 1987 ASHA Convention, a group of speech–language pathologists gathered to present cases they found difficult to diagnose. This three hour session was so warmly received, Sadanand Singh asked us if we would consider publishing the cases in book form. We were so impressed with the professionalism, clinical expertise and insight of our colleagues, and with the value of the information they imparted, that we agreed. Thirteen cases were presented at ASHA. To these, seven have been added, for a total of twenty case studies that challenge our diagnostic acumen. Together, they serve to underscore the fact that a wide variety of factors have the capacity to, and often do, disrupt human communication processes.

The task of differential diagnosis of communication disorders is threefold. First, we must "get the facts." Next, we must isolate and describe those pertinent to the communication breakdown. Finally, we must synthesize these facts into a meaningful, accurate diagnosis. Successful completion of the differential diagnostic process is an art as well as a science. Indeed, the "master clinician" is both an artist and a scientist, combining clinical insight with a broad spectrum of factual knowledge. After reading these case studies, we can add that the "master clinician" also combines the natural inquisitiveness of a detective with the dedication of a humanitarian.

In creating this book, we simply asked our colleagues to describe cases that they found difficult to differentially diagnose, but that had an interesting outcome. Despite this rather random sampling, certain common themes emerged and we were able to group the cases into seven sections. Readers will discover, however, that other themes link the cases to those in other sections. For example, although we have grouped together three patients in whom the primary symptom was adult onset of speech dysfluency, two other cases (one head injury and one dementia) also demonstrated dysfluent behaviors as part of their symptom complex. So, while it is possible to "dip into" this book, readers will benefit enormously from reading each section and chapter in the order they appear.

We begin Section I with Robert Brookshire's description of a 48-year-old man who was referred with "severe spasmodic stuttering speech." Although this man did have central nervous system pathology, Brookshire questioned whether the fluency disorder had a psychogenic component. The patient's response to treatment resolved the etiological dilemma.

Joseph Duffy was asked to see a 50-year-old man with adult onset of stuttering accompanied by secondary behaviors. In addition, his speech was dysprosodic and dysphonic. He had several physical complaints that were potentially neurogenic in origin. Duffy reviews the six clinical observations that led to correct diagnosis and management of this case.

Palilalia (whole word and phrase repetition) is another form of speech dysfluency. Leonard LaPointe describes a 29-year-old man with a history of drug abuse who developed severe palilalia. LaPointe remembered briefly seeing a similar case some years before, and used this new opportunity to carefully delineate the speech patterns of this fascinating communication disorder.

In Section II, the reader will find two head injury cases in which diagnosis and management of the communication problems were complicated by unusual psychological behaviors. Michael Collins discusses the case of a 26-year-old man who developed highly inconsistent speech and language problems two years after a motor vehicle accident. At the same time, he was becoming progressively more hostile. Collins used a standardized aphasia test and the patient's behavioral history to determine whether the language problem was organic in nature.

The 34-year-old woman described by Brenda Adamovich sustained a severe closed-head injury in an auto accident. As she recovered physically and cognitively, a number of bizarre behaviors developed that disrupted her rehabilitation program. The etiology of these behaviors was unclear, but the diagnostic choices included a frontal lobe syndrome, an attentional disorder, mental illness, and normal reaction to mental stress. Adamovich addresses each of these possibilities, thus providing us with valuable differential diagnostic information.

The four cases presented in Section III have several things in common. First, all were men who were either 67 or 68 years of age when they were referred to speech–language pathology. Second, all originally were thought by medical staff to be either "crazy," "drunk," or "malingering." Third, none had a previous history of psychological or psychiatric problems. Fourth, all were subsequently shown to have a neurogenic communication problem. We point this out because the lesson appears to be that when an older adult develops sudden onset of communication problems, a neurological etiology should be the initial consideration. The first case in point is discussed by Jon Lyon. He was asked to see a 67-year-old man whose major behavioral sign was a 5 to 12 second delay before initiating any purposeful, communicative response. Although the patient appeared to be fully cooperative and willing to participate in the language exam, Lyon was forced to consider a psychogenic, as well as a physiological, basis for the behavior. His conclusion has interesting theoretical implications.

The case described by Felice Loverso and Lyanne Riley is, perhaps, the most unusual in the series. Although their patient had no fixed brain lesion, he showed intermittent signs of the relatively rare syndrome of pure-word deafness. The intermittent nature of the disorder forced the question of a functional etiology. The medical history was important to the final diagnosis.

James Aten received a consult on a 67-year-old man who came to the Emergency Room "acting agitated and confused with aggressive and paranoid tendencies — speaking and acting bizzarely." Subsequently, he was taken to a locked psychiatric ward before a physician thought of obtaining the opinion of a Speech and Language Pathologist. The patient was found to have a well-known form of aphasia.

In a similar case, Nancy Drew saw a 68-year-old man who "appeared to be drunk" when admitted to the hospital. Later, physicians decided that he was severely aphasic, but no differential diagnosis as to the type of aphasia was made because the lesion site was not compatible with the "best-fit" syndrome, that is, Wernicke's aphasia. Drew, however, is able to explain the language behaviors on the basis of lesion location.

Section IV groups two cases in which the differential diagnosis of aphasia is complicated by visuospatial disturbances. We begin with the case of a 61-year-old male seen by Leslie Gonzalez-Rothi and Todd Feinberg. In addition to displaying memory problems and a visual field deficit, the patient showed neglect, hemiparesis, apraxia, and a type of aphasia not explained by his posterior cerebral artery stroke. It was found that a multimodal associated agnosia resulted in language test scores that were misinterpreted as typical of transcortical sensory aphasia. Gonzalez-Rothi and Feinberg point out that it is important to identify the underlying mechanisms responsible for poor test results if a patient is to be successfully rehabilitated.

The 67-year-old man described by Kevin Kearns and Katherine Yedor was referred for an aphasia evaluation. Careful examination showed that he had an "optic aphasia" which interfered with correct response to visual test stimuli. This case reminds us that we must look at the patient's behavior en route to a solution, and not just at the final test scores.

In Section V, readers will find three cases in which atypical speech and language problems complicated the classification of aphasia even for these highly experienced clinicians. John Rosenbek, Ross Levine, and Jo Anne Robbins were puzzled by the language behavior of a 67-year-old man who was said to have experienced a left, middle cerebral artery stroke. The hallmark of his verbal expression was great variability, with hypophonic, monotonous, and dyscoordinated qualities. These and other behaviors were eventually found to be predictable sequelae of what was actually a posterior cerebral artery infarction.

The diagnostic question posed by the 64-year-old woman seen by Robert

Wertz, Ellen Bernstein-Ellis, and Jan Roberts is whether this woman had conduction aphasia or (as reported by another clinician) aphasia with apraxia of speech. These clinicians used a therapy approach in solving this not uncommon diagnostic problem. They explain how this approach helped them reach a conclusion.

The 57-year-old man seen by Thomas Prescott showed an unusual pattern of language deficits, the most striking of which was his ability to repeat sentences but not single words in the face of marked auditory comprehension problems. In addition, he far exceeded the language recovery predicted by a standardized aphasia test. Prescott reviews the pertinent literature in helping us unravel this puzzling case.

With the two cases presented in Section VI readers will experience a nice change of pace. Language was not an issue in either case, although both women had a notable communication problem. First, Christy Ludlow, Susan Sedory, and Mihoko Fujita describe a 61-year-old woman who was referred with a diagnosis of spasmodic dysphonia. Her unusual history and features raised several other diagnostic possibilities. Rather than the laryngeal problems typically associated with spasmodic dysphonia, she was found to have laryngeal and respiratory dystonia. This correct diagnosis led to successful treatment.

Kathryn Yorkston was faced with the problem of predicting the impact of a cosmetic surgical procedure on speech intelligibility. The 32-year-old woman, in this case, had suffered a brain stem stroke that left her with a severe right facial paralysis. By performing a seventh to twelfth cranial nerve anastomosis, the surgeons hoped to improve the young woman's appearance, but loss of innervation to the tongue was expected to increase dysarthria. Yorkston reviews the decision-making process and the results.

Section VII brings together four cases in which speech and language problems preceded other signs of a dementing process. It is our impression that such cases may represent an expanding segment of our clinical population, and that these descriptions of dementia subtypes will assist us all in making differential diagnoses. Kathryn Bayles and Cheryl Tomoeda begin the section by describing a 68-year-old man who had recovered from a stroke eight years before being seen for questionable behavioral decline. Because this patient had been seen as an aphasic patient as part of a research project over five years earlier, he presented a unique opportunity to study and compare aphasia versus dementia. The differential diagnostic process as outlined by Bayles and Tomoeda provides readers with a valuable clinical guide.

The 69-year-old woman referred to Jennifer Horner and John Riski had developed signs of aphasia, alexia, agraphia, apraxia of speech and limb, and dysarthria with dysphonia and dysprosodia. In addition, she showed progressive cognitive decline. All of these behaviors occurred in the context of a normal MRI, EEG, and EMG. Horner and Riski present five possible diagnoses and identify issues worthy of future research.

Audrey Holland reviews the case of a 76-year-old man in which the diagnosis of Pick's disease is confirmed by a neuropathological report. Although this case has been described elsewhere, Holland presents us with the rare opportunity to follow along with a master clinician as she solves this diagnostic problem while, at the same time, assisting the patient and his family through this difficult period.

In the concluding chapter, Nancy Helm-Estabrooks, Marjorie Nicholas, and Alisa Morgan present a case that represents a review of many of the diagnostic issues raised by other cases. Their patient was a 52-year-old man with a rather complicated medical and vocational history when referred for "stammering speech." The referring physician raised the question of stroke, although a previous physician had attributed the decline in writing skills to Parkinson's disease. In addition to the stuttering-like behavior and severe dysgraphia, the patient was palilalic and aphasic, with noted set and attentional problems. Helm-Estabrooks, Nicholas, and Morgan discuss six syndromes that might account for the patient's constellation of symptoms.

In closing, we once again underscore the fact that human communication is subject to a variety of influences, and the manifestations of these influences appear infinite. Not infrequently, we are asked to solve diagnostic puzzles. Sometimes, the puzzle is never solved. We believe, however, that by sharing these cases, we all can improve our diagnostic and management skills for the ultimate benefit of our patients.

Nancy Helm-Estabrooks
Boston, Massachusetts

James L. Aten
Long Beach, California

CONTRIBUTORS

Brenda B. Adamovich, Ph.D.
Regional Rehabilitation Center
Mercy Hospital
Springfield, Massachusetts

James L. Aten, Ph.D.
Audiology/Speech Pathology Service
VA Medical Center
Long Beach, California

Kathryn A. Bayles, Ph.D.
Department of Speech & Hearing Sciences
University of Arizona
Tucson, Arizona

Ellen G. Bernstein-Ellis, M.A.
Audiology/Speech Pathology Service
VA Medical Center
Martinez, California

Robert H. Brookshire, Ph.D.
Speech Pathology Section
Neurology Service
VA Medical Center
Minneapolis, Minnesota

Michael Collins, Ph.D.
Audiology/Speech Pathology Service
VA Medical Center
Madison, Wisconsin

Nancy Drew, M.A.
Audiology/Speech Pathology Service
VA Medical Center
San Francisco, California

Joseph R. Duffy, Ph.D.
Speech Pathology Section
Department of Neurology
Mayo Clinic
Rochester, Minnesota

Todd E. Feinberg, M.D.
Neurology Service
VA Medical Center
Gainesville, Florida

Mihoko Fujita, M.D.
Speech & Voice Unit
Human Motor Control Section
MNB-NINCDS, National Institutes of Health
Bethesda, Maryland

Leslie Gonzalez-Rothi, Ph.D.
Audiology/Speech Pathology Service
VA Medical Center
Gainesville, Florida

Nancy Helm-Estabrooks, Sc.D.
Audiology/Speech Pathology Service
VA Medical Center
Boston, Massachusetts

Audrey L. Holland, Ph.D.
Center for Speech/Language/Voice Pathology
Eye and Ear Hospital of Pittsburgh
Pittsburgh, Pennsylvania

Jennifer Horner, Ph.D.
Department of Surgery
Duke University Medical Center
Durham, North Carolina

Kevin P. Kearns, Ph.D.
Audiology/Speech Pathology Service
VA Medical Center
North Chicago, Illinois

Leonard LaPointe, Ph.D.
Department of Speech
   & Hearing Sciences
Arizona State University
Tempe, Arizona

Ross Levine, M.D.
Department of Neurology
University of Wisconsin Medical Center
Madison, Wisconsin

Felice L. Loverso, Ph.D.
Audiology/Speech Pathology Service
VA Medical Center
Columbia, Missouri

Christy L. Ludlow, Ph.D.
Speech & Voice Unit
Human Motor Control Section
MNB-NINCDS, National Institutes of Health
Bethesda, Maryland

Jon G. Lyon, Ph.D.
Speech Pathology Section
Rehabilitative Medicine
VA Medical Center
Reno, Nevada

Alisa Morgan, Ph.D.
Audiology/Speech Pathology Service
VA Medical Center
Boston, Massachusetts

Marjorie Nicholas, M.S.
Audiology/Speech Pathology Service
VA Medical Center
Boston, Massachusetts

Thomas E. Prescott, Ph.D.
Audiology/Speech Pathology Service
VA Medical Center
Denver, Colorado

Lyanne Riley, M.A.
Audiology/Speech Pathology Service
VA Medical Center
Columbia, Missouri

John E. Riski, M.D.
Department of Surgery
Duke University Medical Center
Durham, North Carolina

Jo Anne Robbins, Ph.D.
Department of Neurology
University of Wisconsin Medical Center
Madison, Wisconsin

Jan A. Roberts, Ph.D.
Audiology/Speech Pathology Service
VA Medical Center
Martinez, California

John C. Rosenbek, Ph.D.
Audiology/Speech Pathology Service
VA Medical Center
Madison, Wisconsin

Susan E. Sedory, M.A.
Speech & Voice Unit
Human Motor Control Section
MNB-NINCDS, National Institutes of Health
Bethesda, Maryland

Cheryl K. Tomoeda, M.S.
Department of Speech & Hearing Sciences
University of Arizona
Tucson, Arizona

Robert T. Wertz, Ph.D.
Audiology/Speech Pathology Service
VA Medical Center
Martinez, California

Katherine Yedor, M.A.
Audiology/Speech Pathology Service
VA Medical Center
North Chicago, Illinois

Kathryn M. Yorkston, Ph.D.
Speech Pathology Service
Department of Rehabilitative Medicine
University of Washington
Seattle, Washington

SECTION I

QUESTION OF
NEUROGENIC ETIOLOGY
IN ADULTS WITH
ACQUIRED FLUENCY
DISORDERS

Chapter 1

Robert H. Brookshire

████████████████████

A Dramatic Response to Behavior Modification by a Patient with Rapid Onset of Dysfluent Speech

Background

J.C. was a 48-year-old man who had worked as a materials supervisor for a small construction company prior to a cerebrovascular accident (CVA) nine months before admission to the Minneapolis Veterans Administration Medical Center (VAMC). He had been married, but was divorced several years before his CVA. At the time of his CVA he was living with his parents. He was referred to Speech Pathology Section by Neurology Service for evaluation of "severe spasmodic stuttering speech."

J.C. was first interviewed at bedside. He was alert, cooperative, and oriented to time, place, and person. His comprehension appeared normal for conversation. His spontaneous speech appeared normal in grammatic and semantic content, but was markedly dysfluent, with effortful phonation, repetition of sounds and syllables; grimacing, and exaggerated articulatory movements.

He reported that he had had "a stroke" nine months before, with slowly resolving paralysis of his right arm and leg. He now reported residual weakness, but could walk with a leg brace, and he ate and wrote with his right (preferred) hand. He reported moderate word retrieval problems during the first few weeks following the stroke, but these problems had essentially disappeared by four or five weeks after the stroke. Four months before admission to VAMC he began to notice problems with vision in his right eye, and worsening speech. The visual problem eventually resolved, but his speech continued to deteriorate. During the month preceding his admission he noticed increasing problems with word retrieval, memory, and concentration. He reported that the facial weakness, memory problems, and concentration problems had essentially resolved, but that his speech was still deteriorating.

MEDICAL HISTORY AND NEUROLOGIC EXAMINATION

J.C.'s medical history was relatively complex. He reported a severe streptococcal infection eight years prior to admission, which lasted for several weeks before responding to antibiotics prescribed by his personal physician. Five years before his admission, an intestinal bypass operation was performed at the University of Minnesota to resolve massive obesity. Following surgery, J.C.'s weight decreased from over 300 pounds to the 180s. There were no apparent complications, except for occasional bouts of diarrhea and a period of low-level anemia, both corrected with medications. J.C. denied neurologic, cognitive, or linguistic manifestations of surgery or its aftermath. No medical records concerning any of these events were available, including J.C.'s report of a left-hemisphere CVA nine months earlier.

J.C. reported that he had been a chronic alcoholic, but that he had stopped excessive use of alcohol at the time of his intestinal bypass. He had received medications from his personal physician for several episodes of severe depression "four or five times" during the preceding 10 years, the last approximately 18 months before his CVA. He did not remember the names of the medications or their dosages. He reported that he had never taken such medications for more than a few weeks, that they seemed to help his depression, and that he noticed no side effects while he was taking them.

J.C.'s neurologic examination was generally consistent with his history. He exhibited right central VIIth nerve paresis, mild right hemiparesis and hemianesthesia, and slightly exaggerated deep tendon reflexes on his right side. Cranial nerves other than the VIIth nerve were functionally normal. Muscle masses were within normal limits, with no fasciculations noted. Tests for cerebellar function were within normal limits, except for moderate reductions in rapid limb and tongue movements, which could not be localized specifically to the cerebellum. Gait was normal, except for circumduction of the right hip. The examining neurologist noted that J.C.'s right-sided limb weakness "may be exaggerated by lack of volitional effort," and noted the possible presence of a "psychiatric overlay." However, he concluded, "the patient does have bona fide neurologic disease — etiology unknown."

A comprehensive follow-up neurologic examination was requested to better define the neurologic reasons for J.C.'s speech disorder. The results of this examination were generally consistent with those of the first, except that "choreiform movements"* of J.C.'s tongue and outstretched hands were reported. Dysmetria in repetitive movements of oral structures, wrists, hands, and fingers was present. The neurologic diagnosis following this examination was "probable choreiform state." A CT scan and laboratory tests to rule out Wilson's disease and heavy metal toxicity were ordered. The CT scan (with contrast) revealed no enhancing lesions in either hemisphere, and the results of lab tests for Wilson's disease and heavy metal poisoning were negative. The examining neurologist commented that J.C.'s "choreiform state" probably would progress, with consequent worsening of his speech dysfluency.

SPEECH AND LANGUAGE EVALUATION

The Porch Index of Communicative Ability (PICA) (Porch, 1967) was administered. J.C.'s overall PICA score was 13.05, which placed him at the 81st percentile for aphasic adults. His gestural, verbal, and graphic scores (and percentiles) were 14.11 (84), 12.45 (58), and 12.03 (87), respectively. Verbal responses were delayed, distorted, and/or incomplete, but grammatically and semantically appropriate. J.C.'s deficiencies on the PICA appeared to be related to his speech production difficulties and did not appear to represent language disability. On the 62-item version of the Token Test (DeRenzi & Vignolo, 1962), J.C. made two errors, indicating that his comprehension of spoken directions was within normal limits. On the Word Fluency Measure (Borkowski, Benton, & Spreen, 1967) J.C. produced 38 words. This score placed him at the 10th percentile for adults his age and probably was a consequence of his speech production difficulties. On the

---

*J.C.'s involuntary tongue movements resemble in some respects those described in an unusual disorder called palatal myoclonus, which is characterized by slow (60 to 100 cycles per minute) involuntary movements of the soft palate, pharynx, facial muscles, tongue, and vocal folds, or some combination thereof. Palatal myoclonus is caused by degeneration of the olivary complex in the brain stem. Adams & Victor (1981) assert that this syndrome should not be called myoclonic, because it has little in common with other myoclonic syndromes. It seems doubtful that J.C.'s case represented palatal myoclonus because his hands were also dyskinesic, and because he had no other signs of brain stem involvement.

Nelson Reading Test (Nelson, 1962) J.C. obtained a reading grade level of 7.6, which was considered consistent with his educational and vocational background.

Nonspeech oral movements were generally slow and effortful. Volitional tongue movements appeared especially involved, with slow, clumsy side-to-side movement and restricted tongue-tip elevation. Myoclonic tongue movements were present at rest. Phonation was strained and effortful. J.C. could sustain vowel phonation for no more than four seconds, because of apparently uncontrollable contraction of laryngeal muscles. There was a striking visible increase in J.C.'s general level of muscle tension whenever he attempted to speak; if he was sitting, this tension sometimes caused contractions strong enough to lift one or both feet from the floor. Right-sided facial signs, consistent with VIIth nerve involvement, were present. Oral reading and singing, both alone and in unison with the examiner, were slow and effortful and not perceptibly different from J.C.'s spontaneous speech.

CONCLUSIONS AND RECOMMENDATIONS

ETIOLOGY OF J.C.'S SPEECH DYSFLUENCY

Several potential sources of J.C.'s speech dysfluency were considered.

SEQUELAE OF CVA NINE MONTHS EARLIER

We first considered the possibility that J.C.'s speech dysfluency had its source in the CVA that reportedly had occurred nine months earlier. However, the following observations argued against such a conclusion.

1. J.C.'s speech disturbance had resolved by four or five weeks post-stroke, with sudden worsening several months later. One rarely sees sudden exacerbation of symptoms during uncomplicated recovery from CVA, especially several months later.

2. J.C.'s language was, as far as we could determine, normal. One would expect measurable language impairment, given a left-hemisphere lesion sufficient to disrupt speech to the degree exhibited by J.C.

3. Laboratory and radiologic tests were negative with respect to central nervous system pathology.

4. Dyskinesias such as those exhibited by J.C. are usually associated with extrapyramidal disease, rather than with cortical or subcortical lesions, which typically cause aphasia. A deep lesion could conceivably cause aphasia and dyskinesia, but deep lesions almost always cause dense hemiplegia, which

does not resolve. J.C.'s mild hemiparesis was not consistent with a deep cerebral lesion sufficient to generate the symptoms observed.

A SECOND CEREBROVASCULAR ACCIDENT

The sudden appearance of J.C.'s speech dysfluency and other mental anomalies might have been caused by a second CVA. This conclusion seemed unlikely, for reasons 2, 3, and 4.

TARDIVE DYSKINESIA

Some medications prescribed for amelioration of depression have been shown to produce dyskinesias, particularly when administered at high dosage levels and for long periods of time (Fann, Smith, Davis, & Domino, 1982). This seemed an unlikely source for J.C.'s dysfluency, because his antidepressive medication had been discontinuous and low-dose, and had been terminated well before the onset of J.C.'s dysfluency. Furthermore, tardive dyskinesia usually is characterized by involuntary movements, such as lip-smacking and chewing, in the absence of volitional effort. J.C. produced no such movements.

PSYCHOGENIC DYSFLUENCY

It seemed possible that J.C.'s speech dysfluency was psychogenic. J.C. reported a history of depression severe enough to require medication. Various somatic and mental aberrations spontaneously appeared and subsided. Laboratory and radiologic test results did not confirm central nervous system pathology. The admitting neurologist commented on J.C.'s lack of volitional effort during the physical examination. However, no substantial life stresses were obvious, and there was no evidence of secondary gains for J.C. in his dysfluency. J.C.'s personality and general attitude did not suggest that he was malingering. He appeared genuinely concerned and constructively motivated to do something about his speech dysfluency. He did not give the impression of a hysterical personality.

EXTRAPYRAMIDAL DISEASE

The presence of dyskinesia is usually considered indicative of extrapyramidal disease. J.C.'s tongue and hand dyskinesia were consistent with such a diagnosis. Arguing against such a diagnosis, however, were

• All laboratory tests were negative with respect to the presence of central nervous system disease. However, such negative results are not unusual in extrapyramidal disease, particularly early in its course.

• The sudden onset and apparent stabilization of motor symptoms. Extrapyramidal disease usually is characterized by gradual onset and slow exacerbation, although periods of stabilization and even remission sometimes occur.

Conclusions

After considering these potential explanations for J.C.'s symptoms, we adopted the following hypothesis. J.C.'s myoclonic movements and dyskinesia probably were caused by extrapyramidal disease, of which the etiology, onset, and nature are unknown. It seemed possible that low-level symptoms generated by the disease may have been present but unnoticed by J.C. before his CVA. The CVA and subsequent problems with word retrieval and speech may have caused J.C. to be more concerned about speaking and more attentive to minor disruptions of speech. The combination of (1) increased concern about speech and (2) low-level dyskinesia may have led to exaggerated muscle tension when J.C. attempted to speak, creating the dysfluency we now observed. If this hypothesis were correct, it seemed reasonable that we might decrease J.C.'s dysfluency by decreasing his overall level of muscle tension in speech activities. Therefore, J.C. was enrolled in a treatment program that focused on (1) general muscle relaxation, (2) relaxation of speech muscle groups before phonation, and (3) creation of fluent speech by means of a combination of breath control, rate control, and prolongation of vowels and continuant consonants.

Treatment

A variety of techniques for obtaining muscle relaxation and achieving fluent speech were carried out, and J.C. began a commercial taperecorded relaxation training program. By the seventh treatment session J.C. could read 6- to 10-word phrases and sentences aloud without appreciable articulatory or phonatory effort, but at very slow rates (50 to 80 words per minute). By the twelfth session he could converse with the clinician with minimal effort by speaking at the same very slow rate. He was unable to produce fluent rate-controlled speech outside the treatment room under any circumstances. After 21 sessions J.C. had slightly increased his rate of fluent speech in treatment sessions (70 to 90 words per minute), but no extension of fluent speech to interactions outside treatment activities was observed.

Because J.C.'s progress seemed to be slowing, and because little generalization beyond the treatment room had been obtained, we decided to attack his overall level of muscle tension with behavior modification procedures. Because J.C.'s dysfluent speech behaviors were always preceded by general muscle tensing, we hypothesized that we might decrease his dysfluency if we could decrease or prevent anticipatory muscle tensing.

First we constructed a manipulandum consisting of two momentary-contact pushbuttons mounted in each end of a plastic cylinder 1.75 inches long with a 1 inch diameter (Figure 1-1). The pushbuttons were connected in parallel to an electronic timer. The timer was connected to a red indicator light so that when the timer was activated the light came on and remained illuminated for 30 seconds.

We began behavior modification in the twenty-second treatment session. The red indicator light was placed so that it was visible to both J.C. and the clinician, and the manipulandum was placed in J.C.'s right hand, with his thumb on one pushbutton and his forefinger on the other. The operation of the manipulandum-timer-light combination was demonstrated, and J.C. was told that he could say whatever he wished, in any manner that he chose, but that he could not attempt to say anything while the red light was on. J.C. and the clinician then began conversing. On J.C.'s first several attempts at speech his anticipatory muscle tensing caused him to activate the pushbuttons and the light came on before he could initiate phonation. On his nineteenth attempt J.C. said one word (without effort) before muscle tensing caused the light to come on. Throughout the remainder of the session, J.C.'s fluent speech output increased rapidly. By the end of the session he was producing complete sentences fluently and without effort. A brief examination at the end of the session showed that myoclonic tongue movements and hand dyskinesia were present and unchanged. To test the generalization of J.C.'s fluency, he was taken from the treatment room (without the manipulandum) and placed in conversations with the clinic secretary and another speech–language pathologist. His speech remained

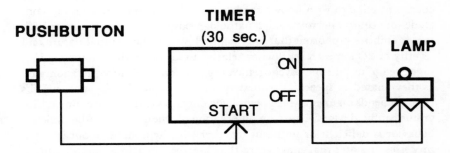

Figure 1-1. A manipulandum consisting of two momentary-contact pushbuttons mounted in each end of a plastic cylinder 1.75 inches long with a 1 inch diameter.

fluent, with occasional short-duration interruptions. Grimacing, glottal tension, and general muscle tension were markedly reduced.

When J.C. returned for his next appointment, his speech was essentially as it had been when he left the clinic three days before. He reported that he had continued to speak fluently in his daily life. When placed in the behavior modification condition J.C. was interrupted by the light four times in the first six minutes. In the remaining 34 minutes of the session he spoke fluently, without effort, and was never interrupted by the light. He and the clinician then left the clinic room and initiated conversations with a number of others, most of them strangers to J.C. His speech was completely fluent and normal.

J.C. reported to the clinic weekly for five weeks. His speech remained fluent and effortless, but his dyskinesic tongue and hand movements remained unchanged. He was then discharged from treatment. We continued to see J.C. occasionally for about eight years following his discharge. His speech remained completely normal in fluency. His dyskinesic tongue and hand movements remained unchanged, and his neurologic condition neither deteriorated nor improved.

DISCUSSION

J.C.'s case is not unusual, in terms of our inability to make a conclusive diagnosis about the causes of his speech abnormalities. Like J.C., many patients arrive at neurologists' offices and examining rooms with behavioral, mental, or affective anomalies apparently caused by nervous system disruptions, but with no objective evidence of such disruptions. In many such cases the major question becomes whether the patient's symptoms are neurogenic or psychogenic in nature. The results of J.C.'s neurologic examination were consistent enough with known syndromes to lead two neurologists to conclude that central nervous system pathology existed. Our own testing of J.C.'s motor abilities supported that judgment. However, the unusual nature and severity of J.C.'s speech dysfluency relative to his nonverbal motor abilities suggested to us possible psychogenic exaggeration of his motoric anomalies as they related to speech. Fortunately, management of cases such as J.C.'s rarely depends on unequivocal neurologic diagnosis. Effective treatment programs can be devised, based on observation of when and how the patient's behavior is deficient or unusual, together with hypotheses about internal processes or states that may create the observed behavioral abnormalities. A positive response to treatment increases the speech–language pathologist's confidence that she or he has guessed right about the underlying internal processes, but absolute certainty is seldom, if ever, the case.

J.C.'s failure at first to achieve fluency beyond the confines of the room in which treatment took place also is not unusual. One of the major therapeutic problems faced by speech–language pathologists, regardless of the disorder being treated, is extension of improvements obtained in treatment sessions to the world outside the treatment room. Our initial procedures were sufficient to produce some degree of fluency in carefully controlled circumstances, but they were not sufficient to extend that fluency to daily life. Placing consistent and inescapable contingencies on behaviors that preceded dysfluent speech generated immediate, dramatic, and durable effects on J.C.'s fluency. Such an approach is not new. Treatment of stuttering has for many years included attention to behaviors or internal states that lead up to stuttering incidents themselves, and this writer (Brookshire, 1970) eliminated supposedly uncontrollable "pseudobulbar crying" in a patient with multiple sclerosis by eliminating head aversion behavior that consistently preceded the crying.

That J.C.'s dysfluency disappeared so quickly in response to behavior modification procedures supports our hypothesis that his dysfluency was in large part psychogenic. Positive response to behavioral treatment is not, of course, definitive with regard to the organic or nonorganic nature of a behavior. However, precipitous elimination of pathologic behavior with initiation of treatment or with changes in a treatment regimen substantially increases the likelihood that the behavior is, to an important extent, psychogenic. To say that J.C.'s dysfluency was psychogenic is not, of course, equivalent to saying that it was intentional on J.C.'s part, or that it should be taken less seriously than if the condition were organic. J.C.'s dysfluency caused him great anxiety, frustration, and unhappiness, and seriously compromised his interactions with others. It was exceedingly "real" to J.C. and to those around him.

J.C.'s response to treatment suggests that he was not malingering. His dysfluency resolved rapidly and completely given appropriate contingencies. The symptoms did not recur, and he developed no substitute symptoms during the eight years that we followed him. We were successful in treating his symptoms even though we were uncertain about their origin, and our success had dramatic and durable effects on J.C.'s life.

REFERENCES

Adams, R.A., & Victor, M. (1981). *Principles of neurology* (2nd ed.). New York: McGraw-Hill.

Borkowski, J.G., Benton, A.L., & Spreen, O. (1967). Word fluency and brain damage. *Neuropsychologia, 5*, 135-140.

Brookshire, R. (1970). Control of "involuntary" crying behavior emitted by a multiple sclerosis patient. *Journal of Communication Disorders, 3,* 171-176.

DeRenzi, E., & Vignolo, L.A. (1962). The token test: A sensitive test to detect receptive disturbances in aphasics. *Brain, 85,* 665-678.

Fann, W.E., Smith, R.C., Davis, J.M., & Domino, E.F. (1982). *Tardive dyskinesia: Research and treatment.* New York: SP Scientific and Medical Books.

Nelson, M.J. (1962). *The Nelson reading test.* New York: Houghton Mifflin.

Porch, B.E. (1967). *Porch index of communicative ability.* Palo Alto, CA: Consulting Psychologists Press.

CHAPTER 2

JOSEPH R. DUFFY

A PUZZLING CASE OF
ADULT ONSET
STUTTERING

*T*his case was referred to Speech Pathology by a staff neurologist who wanted an opinion about the etiology of the patient's speech disturbance. The diagnostic challenge was to establish the probable cause of a speech disturbance that appeared in a context of a more pervasive "illness," in which psychogenic, neurogenic, and other organic factors needed to be addressed. The case has something to teach us about the differential diagnosis of acquired speech disturbances, as well as its role in the comprehensive diagnosis, understanding, and management of human illness.

THE CASE

BRIEF HISTORY

W.H. was a 50-year-old, right-handed, college-educated secretary/treasurer of an oil company. On a questionnaire completed prior to his initial evaluation in the Department of Medicine, he gave the following reason for coming to the Clinic: "Chest pains and inability to speak accompanied by spasms of neck and head." He wrote that his main symptoms were "pronounced stuttering with persistent jerking of head and neck; chest pains persist even though on medicine."

W.H. told the internist of an 18-month history of epigastric and right-upper-quadrant chest pain, which radiated to his neck, teeth, and back.

Shortly after the onset of his pain a coronary catheterization was scheduled to investigate possible cardiac sources. A day or two before that procedure he developed "stuttering spastic speech" and "muscle spasms" in his neck. These lasted several days and remitted, only to return periodically and unpredictably, and with progressively shorter periods of remission. His last remission had lasted for a month. His speech problem was unremitting for the preceding four to five weeks and was present on examination.

During the same 18-month period he also had occasional "trembling" in his hands, abnormal gait, dizziness when standing, and numbness in his hands and feet. He also complained of frequent headaches.

W.H. wanted to know "if there's anything physically wrong with me." His wife was concerned that heart disease or a stroke had caused his symptoms.

GENERAL MEDICAL EXAMINATION

Physical examination was normal except for epigastric and right abdominal tenderness, left anterior tibial dermatitis, and what the internist described as "dystonic speech with head and neck flexion movements." Cardiac and gastroenterology workups were scheduled. Regarding the speech deficit the internist wrote: "Don't know etiology. Neuro consult." He also suspected that W.H. was depressed and arranged for psychiatric consultation.

Over the course of W.H.'s evaluation the following tests were conducted and found to be normal: chest, colon, and kidney x-rays; electrocardiogram; coronary angiogram; and ultrasound of the gallbladder. Extensive laboratory blood tests and urinalysis were unremarkable. Stomach x-ray showed postoperative changes associated with an old diaphragmatic hernia repair; there was a small diaphragmatic hernia. Frequent blood pressure checks were normal.

Additional cardiac tests showed some narrowing of the coronary arteries, but there were no electrocardiographic changes. The cardiologist concluded that there was no evidence of heart disease.

The gastroenterologist recommended liberal use of antacids and elevation of the head during sleep for relief of his epigastric pain.

NEUROLOGICAL EXAMINATION

Neurological examination was conducted on the second day of the workup. The neurologist described W.H.'s speech as "dysphonic and stuttering," with associated platysma contractions. Muscle strength, cranial nerve function, gait, coordination, sensation, and reflexes were normal. Other than the abnormal speech and speech-associated movements, there was no evidence of a movement disorder.

The neurologist thought the speech problem was "most likely a manifestation of tension and perhaps of somatization tendencies, and probably not a manifestation of a cerebellar, basal ganglia, or corticobulbar tract abnormality." He scheduled a CT scan of the head (which was negative) and referred W.H. to Speech Pathology for an opinion about the neurogenic versus psychogenic etiology of the speech disturbance.

Speech Pathology Examination

The speech evaluation was conducted following the neurology consultation. In addition to the history he gave to the intern and neurologist, W.H. indicated that since the first episode of speech disturbance he could anticipate recurrences about two days in advance. He could not anticipate remissions. He said his speech was better in relaxed situations and usually worst at work. He denied chewing or swallowing difficulty. When asked what he believed the etiology of his speech problem was, he said he has not sure, but that it might be related to his feelings of depression, tension, and anxiety. He stated, however, that his wife believed there was an organic explanation. He became teary-eyed on several occasions when relating the history.

W.H.'s conversational speech and reading contained numerous sound and syllable prolongations, repetitions, and hesitations. Rate was moderately slowed, even during phrases in which speech was relatively fluent. Dysfluencies were consistently accompanied by a variety of easily observable movements, which included neck hyperextension, simultaneous retraction of lower face muscles and platysmas, lip pursing, and raising of his eyebrows. These movements were present only during speech. Vocal loudness was mildly to moderately reduced, although W.H. stated that he had always been soft spoken. The prosody of his speech was "flat" beyond what was directly attributable to his dysfluencies. Frequency of dysfluencies fluctuated during conversation, and several utterances were nearly normally fluent. His posture, general body movement, and facial expression were slow, unanimated, and "flat." Together with reduced speech prosody, they conveyed an affect of "depression."

There was no evidence of language impairment. In addition, there were no sound substitutions, omissions, or additions, nor, in spite of his dysfluencies, was there any off-target, audible or visible groping for articulatory postures. No findings supported the diagnosis of apraxia of speech.

His prolongation of "ah" was steady and normal in quality. Alternating motion rates (AMRs) for "puh" and "tuh" were normal; AMRs for "kuh" were mildly irregular and associated with some of the musculoskeletal struggle noted during connected speech.

The lower face, jaw, tongue, and palate were normal in size, strength, symmetry, and range of movement. Gag reflex was normal. Voluntary cough and glottal coup were normal, as were reflexive cough and laugh. There was no sucking reflex and no apparent drooling.

MANAGEMENT OF THE SPEECH DISTURBANCE

At this point it was tentatively concluded that the speech disturbance was predominantly or completely psychogenic in origin. I told W.H. that although the precise reason for the development of his speech difficulty was not yet clear — and might never be — there was no *active* neurological or other organic cause for his current speech symptoms, that he had the potential for normal speech, and that improvement could sometimes be achieved quickly with some hard work. I told him that we could immediately undertake efforts to improve his speech. He agreed to this.

He was told that a major source of his speech dysfluency was the excessive muscular effort and struggle he was exerting in an attempt to speak normally, and that, with less tension and effort, his speech would improve, perhaps dramatically. His platysma contractions were then identified as an example of excessive muscular effort. He was told that on subsequent speech attempts he could excessively contract any muscles *except* his platysmas. He was then asked to read a paragraph. Any excessive platysma contractions were immediately pointed out and he was told to stop and begin again without them. As he read, he was given frequent and immediate encouragement about his progress, and we expressed our optimism that he would continue doing well. Within about five minutes he was no longer excessively contracting his platysmas. We then identified the speech-associated neck hyperextension and went through the same process. At this time all deviant speech characteristics began to improve. Rate increased, and prolongation and repetitions reduced dramatically. After about 20 minutes of this symptomatic work, W.H. spoke normally during reading and conversation for five consecutive minutes. Dysfluencies and associated struggle exhibited thereafter were consistently and dramatically reduced when compared to his presenting disturbance.

When speech improvement was achieved, we talked frankly about the influence of psychological factors on his speech. We discussed the fact that speech disturbances in response to stress, anxiety, anger, and other "negative" emotions are not terribly unusual and can occur in people without serious psychiatric disease. He was told that such problems occur in people who are facing considerable conflict, particularly when the conflict's resolution might require verbal confrontation or expression. W.H. then revealed being greatly dissatisfied with work for several years and said he was struggling with whether or not to leave his well-paying and high-status job for something that was more personally satisfying. He described his marriage as good, but admitted that his wife's insistence that his speech and physical problems were organic, and that he come to our clinic for a comprehensive evaluation, was a source of conflict between them. I expressed the opinion that a complete medical evaluation at this time might put the issue to rest for both of them.

Because of additional scheduled appointments, further symptomatic therapy and discussion of the nature of his speech problem were postponed. Another appointment was scheduled in three days, because of an intervening weekend, and I told him that his speech improvement would probably be maintained over the weekend and that continued improvement was quite possible, especially given his improved insight into the problem.

When next seen, W.H.'s speech was further improved—he said "95 percent normal," and I agreed. He was still aware of some head and neck tension while speaking, but such tension was not observable. Most impressive was a change in his affect. Prosody was near normal, his posture was more upright, and his movements during social interaction were more animated. He looked and sounded very different from the way he had during initial assessment; colleagues who listened to a baseline recording remarked that the post-treatment tape sounded like another person. On this second visit, we spent only a few minutes addressing the remaining speech symptoms, but discussed further the likely connection between his speech problem and the stressful issues in his life. I pointed out that speech difficulties such as his are sometimes maintained as long as their causes are unknown or when physical and neurological explanations are being considered. I stressed that his workup thus far was reassuring insofar as his speech had improved dramatically, his neurological exam was normal, and his cardiac workup was encouraging. He admitted that these findings were removing a major source of anxiety for him, as well as a source of conflict with his wife. He expressed a desire to return home and more directly confront the issues surrounding his work. He admitted that although he had recognized his depression and anxiety, he had until now never appreciated the strong connection between those feelings and his physical symptoms.

I saw W.H. briefly the next day. His speech was normal. He was pleased with his progress. Both of us agreed that there was nothing further to do regarding symptomatic speech therapy. He was encouraged to keep his appointment in Psychiatry.

PSYCHIATRIC EXAMINATION

W.H. was seen in Psychiatry following the final speech appointment. His Minnesota Multiphasic Personality Inventory (MMPI) (Hathaway & McKinley, 1943) showed a response pattern often seen in individuals with functional complaints and conversion disorders. There was a significantly elevated score on the "hypochondriasis" scale, which is sensitive to preoccupation with bodily functions and physical health, frequently without an organic basis. Also significantly elevated was the scale sensitive to "conversion hysteria," or physical symptoms likely to be of hysterical origin.

The psychiatrist established that W.H.'s physical and speech problems usually coincided with increased work load. He felt that W.H. was demoralized by his chronic health problems. Of significance, W.H. reported a 30-year history of brief periods (a few days at most) of severe depression, although these had not occurred in recent years. W.H. admitted that he held on to emotional pain. He again described his marriage as good, but stated that his wife pushed for more medical assessment than he would prefer. The psychiatrist observed that W.H.'s speech was normal, but noted that his affect was "slightly apathetic."

The psychiatrist concluded that there were "psychophysiologic and possible conversion components" present. He noted that while W.H. was able to identify tension and frustration, there was "possible conflict resolution value" of his symptoms in an occupation where he was torn between "fight or leave." The psychiatrist did not believe W.H. was currently suffering from major depression, but might have a cyclic affective disorder; however, he believed W.H.'s cyclic episodes were more strongly tied to personality and stress, and were not endogenous. He also noted that W.H. used minimizing and denial, and that they might be reflected in a tendency toward conversion and depression "out of the blue." He recommended psychotherapy of the supportive/educative type, and biofeedback-assisted feedback training for relaxation. He did not recommend antidepressants. W.H. agreed to follow these recommendations on his return home.

DISCUSSION

The speech diagnosis in this case was stuttering-like behavior of psychogenic origin. It occurred in a person who had a number of physical complaints, several of which were potentially neurological in origin (e.g., the speech problem, numbness, gait complaints, dizziness). Other symptoms required a full cardiac workup, and the cardiac complaints were a potential source of a neurological disturbance (e.g., emboli). As it turned out, neurological and cardiac abnormalities were not identified. Thus, there was no evidence for a neurological basis for W.H.'s speech disturbance and, ultimately, very good evidence that his speech problem was psychogenic. Although speech evaluation and management were sufficient to establish the speech diagnosis, the complete medical workup was essential to the overall understanding of the illness.

Unfortunately, there is an insufficient published data base to permit a listing of signs and symptoms that can be used with confidence to identify the salient and distinguishing features of acquired psychogenic stuttering-like behavior in adults. There are a few published case studies of psychogenic stuttering that are descriptively very informative and provide some clues to its identification and underlying causes (Deal, 1982; Deal & Doro, 1987; Wallen, 1961; Williams, 1978). Careful reading of the literature on acquired neurogenic stuttering, when integrated with the limited data on psychogenic stuttering, contributes further to an appreciation of the clinical features that distinguish between neurogenic and psychogenic stuttering-like behavior. (For comprehensive reviews of adult-onset neurogenic stuttering, see Helm-Estabrooks, 1986, and Rosenbek, 1984).

One thing is clear. Stuttering-like behavior can develop in adults in the absence of neurological disease. In a recent unpublished retrospective study, Baumgartner and Duffy (1986) reported on 49 people seen at the Mayo Clinic over about a 10-year period who were diagnosed as having adult onset of psychogenic stuttering-like behavior; none of them had evidence of neurological disease and none had a history of childhood stuttering. Perhaps even more significant, an additional 20 people were identified who had adult onset of psychogenic stuttering-like behavior in the presence of confirmed neurological disease. Thus, adult onset of psychogenic stuttering, while rare, is not extremely rare, and it can occur in the presence or absence of neurological disease. The lesson is that the assignment of a neurogenic etiology to adult-onset stuttering requires careful consideration, even in the presence of confirmed neurological disease. (This is not to suggest that neurogenic stuttering does not exist, or that neurogenic stuttering cannot be present in the absence of other evidence of neurological disease.)

What, specifically, led to the conclusion that W.H.'s speech problem was psychogenic in origin? The following observations and arguments, *taken together*, led to the diagnosis:

1. The problem was present intermittently. Obviously, this does not rule out a number of neurological etiologies (e.g., transient ischemic attacks, multiple sclerosis, seizures). However, the duration of the speech exacerbations would have been unusual for a number of neurogenic etiologies. In addition, the relative absence of other sensory or motor disturbances, and the absence of accompanying aphasia, dysarthria, or apraxia of speech, is not the milieu in which neurogenic stuttering usually appears. Taken together, these observations argue against a neurogenic etiology (but, admittedly, do not rule it out).

2. W.H.'s ability to predict recurrence of the speech problems up to a few days in advance would be rare in neurological disease, and very possibly reflected awareness of increasing psychological stress.

3. The speech problem was, to some degree, event specific; worse at work, better when away from work. This is not to argue that stress and anxiety cannot influence the severity of neurogenic speech disturbances, but the degree to which W.H. was reportedly affected by environmental events seemed extreme for that usually encountered in neurological disease. Such situational variability is not uncommon in functional disorders.

4. The nature of the dysfluencies (repetitions, prolongations, hesitations) do not, in our experience, reliably distinguish neurogenic from psychogenic stuttering (Baumgartner & Duffy, 1986). However, the amount of associated excessive muscular movement and tension does. Such tension and movements were striking in W.H., were present only during speech, and did not resemble those seen in movement disorders such as chorea, athetosis, torticollis, and dystonia. His degree of "secondary struggle" would have been unusual in neurogenic stuttering, but is not uncommon in psychogenic stuttering.

5. W.H. admitted to feelings of depression and unhappiness at work, and his speech and overall affect conveyed an image of depression. His MMPI and psychiatric evaluation were confirmatory of active relevant psychological factors.

6. The most convincing evidence was provided by the treatment results. Assertively but supportively undertaken, without admonishment for having "succumbed" to life's stresses, symptomatic treatment resulted in rapid, dramatic, and lasting (days, at least) speech improvement. To argue that W.H.'s response to treatment was coincident with a remission of a neurogenic disturbance is nearly indefensible, given the continuous presence of his speech problem four to five weeks prior to evaluation. It is of value to note that in Baumgartner and Duffy's (1986) retrospective study approximately 50 percent of the patients with psychogenic stuttering, including those with neurological disease, who were treated improved to normal or near normal in one or two sessions. Not only are such results of significant benefit to the patient, they confirm the diagnosis as psychogenic.

The outcome in this case was good. W.H. went home speaking normally, reassured because of a comprehensive medical workup that he had no serious cardiac or neurological disease. He also had improved insight and understanding that his speech and many of his physical symptoms represented a response to psychological factors, a portion of which was potentially manageable. The speech evaluation, diagnosis, and management contributed to this outcome, perhaps crucially, and demonstrated that speech pathology has something to contribute to medicine beyond the treatment of disorders whose diagnoses are clearly established. More specifically, this case illustrates that

1. Stuttering-like behavior can develop in adulthood
2. It can be psychogenic in origin
3. Psychogenic stuttering-like behavior can occur in people suspected of having neurological disease
4. Psychologically supportive and informative symptomatic therapy sometimes results in rapid and dramatic speech improvement, providing, at the very least, functional relief for the patient, and confirmation of the etiology as psychogenic.

REFERENCES

Baumgartner, J., & Duffy, J.R. (November, 1986). *Adult onset stuttering: psychogenic and/or neurogenic.* Miniseminar presented at American Speech-Language-Hearing Association Convention, Detroit, MI.

Deal, J.L. (1982). Sudden onset of stuttering: A case report. *Journal of Speech and Hearing Disorders, 47,* 301–304.

Deal, J.L., & Doro, J.M. (1987). Episodic hysterical stuttering. *Journal of Speech and Hearing Disorders, 52,* 299–300.

Hathaway, S.R., & McKinley, J.C. (1943). *The Minnesota multiphasic personality inventory.* Minneapolis: University of Minnesota Press.

Helm-Estabrooks, N. (1986). Diagnosis and management of neurogenic stuttering in adults. In K.O. St. Louis (Ed.), *The atypical stutterer: Principles and practices of rehabilitation.* Orlando, FL: Academic Press.

Rosenbek, J.C. (1984). Stuttering secondary to nervous system damage. In R.F. Curlee & W.H. Perkins (Eds.), *Nature and treatment of stuttering: New directions.* San Diego: College-Hill Press.

Wallen, V. (1961). Primary stuttering in a 28-year-old adult. *Journal of Speech and Hearing Disorders, 26,* 394–395.

Williams, D.E. (1978). Differential diagnosis of disorders of fluency. In F.L. Darley & D.C. Spriestersbach (Eds.), *Diagnostic methods in speech pathology.* New York: Harper & Row.

CHAPTER 3

LEONARD L. LAPOINTE

PROGRESSIVE ECHOLALIA AND ECHOPRAXIA: WHAT COULD IT BE? WHAT COULD IT BE?

*A*fter a few years of experience in a typical clinic that specializes in adult neurogenic communication disorders, a clinician can begin to predict with a reasonable degree of accuracy the mix of disorders that will be represented in a weekly case load. An assortment of aphasia types and a few varieties of neuromotor speech disorders is the usual array, perhaps seasoned with an unusual case or two. For the clinician who is challenged by unusual exercise in differential diagnosis, some of the most intriguing clinical questions are presented by those cases that occur only once in a blue moon. While this type of mystery may invigorate the clinician, to the patient who possesses an unusual or challenging disorder, epidemiologic statistics are little comfort. Worry is *not* lessened by the assurance that "this type of disorder is as rare as a real green chili tamale in Ontonagon, Michigan." Worry *is* lessened, however, by the perception that the clinician in charge is thorough, concerned, and well-grounded in the principles of appraisal and diagnosis.

This chapter describes one of those blue-moon differential diagnostic challenges. Also presented are some of the speech behaviors that were collected and studied, and served to further define the characteristics of this unique speech disorder.

Consultation Request and Background

The subject of this report is a 29-year-old man with a four-year history of a puzzling speech disorder, who was referred to our Audiology and Speech Pathology Service at a Veteran's Administration Medical Center.

J.L.B. was referred to us from Psychiatry Service for evaluation of "progressive echolalia and echopraxia." This was his first admission to our hospital, and notes at the time listed complaints of headaches of three-weeks duration, a sleep disorder, and "progressive perseveration of speech" over the past two and one-half years. Hospital notes also reported a gait disturbance referred to as "astasia-abasia," or difficulty in attempts to stand or walk due to motor incoordination.

Psychiatric evaluation reports stated that J.L.B. had suspected but unconfirmed phenobarbital addiction; an admitted history of barbiturate use; remote and flat affect; poor interpersonal relations; and lack of motivation. The tentative diagnostic conclusion of the psychiatric evaluation was that J.L.B.'s problem was "simple schizophrenia."

Perhaps because of the motor incoordination gait problem and the unusual speech pattern, he was referred to Neurology Service for further assessment. Reports of the neurological evaluation indicated no evidence of EEG abnormality. J.L.B. was scheduled for a brain scan, skull films, and further neurodiagnostics, but he left the hospital against medical advice before their completion. Prior to his unexpected and unrecommended departure, we were able to see him over a four-day period.

Speech-Language Evaluation

Our consultation request from Psychiatry Service listed a "29-year-old man with progressive echolalia and echopraxia. Please evaluate." We were able to see him for four two-hour sessions during his brief hospitalization, and fortunately were able to taperecord his speech and language during a variety of communication tasks. In addition, he was administered several standardized communication measures.

Orientation, short-term memory, and auditory comprehension skills were intact, and no aphasic deficit was detected. He achieved an overall Porch Index of Communicative Ability (PICA) (Porch, 1967) score at the eighty-eighth percentile, but this slightly depressed score easily could be accounted for by his slight motoric difficulty, which resulted in mildly distorted writing errors.

REITERATION, REITERATION

The most striking feature of J.L.B.'s speech pattern was apparent only in his verbal output; his speech was marked by obvious and frequent reiteration.

A superlative example of J.L.B.'s verbal production is presented in the following response to the question, "What does 'look before you leap' mean?" His answer:

> You should look, look, look, look in, look in, look in, you should, you should look in, [+52 reiterations] you should, you should, you should look, look, look into, into, into things, things, things before, before, before, before you go, you go, you go into them.

We were curious to explore whether or not the reiteration varied across conditions or speech tasks with this type of dramatic verbal aberration. J.L.B. reported no unusual communicative situations under which the reiteration was significantly altered, with the exception of somewhat more trouble under conditions of fatigue or stress. He was unable to inhibit the reiteration volitionally.

SPEECH TASKS

To further evaluate the type, locus, and frequency of reiterative utterances, we taperecorded his output across seven basic types of tasks. These included:

1. Verbal formulation tasks
    a. "Tell me three things you did today."
    b. Sentence formulation, Subtest C-11 from Schuell's Minnesota Test for the Differential Diagnosis of Aphasia (MTDDA) (Schuell, 1965)
    c. Definitions
    d. Verbalizing a hypothetical situation ("Tell me what you do when your car runs out of gas")
2. Conversational spontaneous speech
3. Picture description
    a. Card 11, Subtest C-12 (MTDDA)
    b. Tornado picture
    c. Cookie theft picture from Boston Diagnostic Aphasia Exam (BDAE) (Goodglass & Kaplan, 1983)
4. Sentence reading
    a. Subtest L, BDAE
    b. Fisher-Logemann test sentences (Fisher & Logemann, 1971)
5. Paragraph reading
    a. Rainbow passage
    b. Grandfather passage

6. Automatic speech (counting, days of week, etc., from BDAE, II, B)
7. Repetition of phrases and sentences
   a. Phrases (BDAE, III, E)
   b. Sentences (Fisher-Logemann)

From J.L.B.'s responses to these tasks, we were able to discover much about both the severity and type of his unusual verbal output disorder. First, relative to severity, it became apparent that nearly half of his speech was plagued by reiteration. In fact, 2,087 reiterations were counted from a total sample of 5,489 words. Thus, 38 percent of J.L.B.'s total recorded speech output was repeated, varying from 1 iteration to a maximum of 52, which occurred in the explanation of the proverb "look before you leap" presented earlier.

Eight types of reiteration became apparent from analysis of the corpus of recorded material across speech tasks. These reiteration types included:

1. One word—"... from the gods to *foretell, foretell, foretell*..."
2. Phrase—"... in the air they act, *they act, they act* like..."
3. Phrase reiterated within reiterated phrase —"... a plump worm, *a plump, a plump,* a plump worm..."
4. Phrase within a phrase—"... let me, *let me* keep a little wedding cake..."
5. Word reiteration within a reiterated phrase —"... of white light, of *white, white* light..."
6. Sentence—"I own a coat. *I own a coat.*"
7. Syllabic element—"... torn-, *torn-,* tornado..."
8. Unintelligible utterance

What Could It Be? What Could It Be?

We were faced with the task of arriving at a speech diagnosis of this puzzling disorder. I had encountered what I recalled vaguely as a similar condition in a patient seen in an armed forces hospital in Denver during the Vietnam war era. This war-injured veteran's output puzzled all of the local experts, and as a graduate student in training, I was no doubt the most baffled. The veteran's response to the question "Where are you from?" was a dramatic, "Hayward, Kansas, Hayward, Kansas, Hayward, Kansas, Hayward, Kansas, Hayward, Kansas..." until he ran out of breath. We arrived at no speech diagnosis, the young man was soon transferred, and the mystery remained unsolved.*

---

*One of editors (J.A.) was among the group of "puzzled experts," but does recall that the patient had a shell fragment located on lateral x-ray as being deep subcortically in the centraencephalon and not resectable.

Now we had anotner. The immediate temptation was to ascribe the condition to one of the dysfluency syndromes. The nature of the speech disruption suggested that this was very unlike the speech repetition and prolongation pattern usually seen in stuttering. We considered what conditions could result in disrupted speech flow and thought of the occasional dysfluencies sometimes heard in the aphasias or neuromotor speech disorders. Other possibilities included perhaps some rare form of adult onset dysfluency syndrome, perhaps echolalia, perhaps a verbal tic disorder such as that seen in Tourette's syndrome. We entertained as well that we might be dealing with one of the neurogenic atypical stuttering patterns such as those described by Farmer (1975) or Helm-Estabrooks (1986).

Speech Diagnosis

Further analysis and familiarity with the quality and severity of J.L.B.'s reiterated verbal output, coupled with careful literature search for similar cases previously described, revealed that this disorder indeed was not unknown; though rare, it had been previously described on several occasions. Several references were found in the literature of patients who were described as presenting speech characterized by reiteration of utterances, usually with an increasing rate and decreasing loudness. This disorder was called *palilalia*, and some characterized it as compulsive reiteration of utterances. While the etiology has never been incontrovertibly revealed, it has been associated with bilateral subcortical neuropathology (Boller, Boller, Denes, Timberlake, Zieper, & Albert, 1973). Brown (1972) suggested that this rare phenomenon was labelled *cataphasia* and *self-echolalia* in the late 1800s, but that the term *palilalia* was introduced by Souques in 1908. Brown (1972) and Boller, Albert, and Denes (1979) outlined some of the general speech characteristics and described its neurophysiologic substrates, but detailed description of the type, locus, and frequency of reiterative utterances across a variety of speech tasks was not presented until 1981 in the *Journal of Speech and Hearing Disorders* (LaPointe & Horner, 1981). This was followed by a further study of the acoustic properties of pathologic reiterative utterances by Kent and LaPointe (1982).

Since the appearance of these detailed case descriptions of palilalia in the early 1980s, the number of clinical anecdotes regarding the presence of palilalia on the case loads of speech–language pathologists throughout the United States appears to suggest that perhaps the condition is not as rare as once suspected. However, there still exists no epidemiologic study on the prevalence or incidence of the disorder, nor are we aware of further clarification of the suggested neuropathology of the disorder by contemporary neuroimaging techniques. The only paper on management of palilalia describes the use of a pacing board to regulate speech output (Helm, 1979).

It does not seem farfetched to suggest that the abundance of rate manipulation strategies suggested for use in the treatment of the dysarthrias (Yorkston, Beukelman, & Bell, 1988) might well be a fruitful avenue to explore with palilalia.

This case taught us much. In addition to the puzzlement that piqued our curiosity and sent us to the clinical literature in search of answers, it also provided the impetus for a series of careful descriptive studies, which extended our ability to differentially diagnose palilalia. Perhaps someday this information can be used to treat more effectively this remarkable disorder.

REFERENCES

Boller, F., Albert, M., & Denes, F. (1979). Palilalia. *British Journal of Disorders of Communication*, *10*, 92–97.

Boller, F., Boller, M., Denes, G., Timberlake, W., Zieper, I., & Albert, M. (1973). Familial palilalia. *Neurology*, *23*, 1117–1125.

Brown, J.W. (1972). *Aphasia, apraxia and agnosia*. Springfield, IL: Charles C. Thomas.

Farmer, A. (1975). Stuttering repetitions in aphasic and nonaphasic brain damaged adults. *Cortex*, *11*, 391–396.

Fisher, H., & Logemann, J.A. (1971). *Fisher-Logemann test of articulation competence*. Boston: Houghton Mifflin.

Goodglass, H., & Kaplan, E. (1983). *Boston diagnostic aphasia examination*. Philadelphia: Lea and Febiger.

Helm, N. (1979). Management of palilalia with a pacing board. *Journal of Speech and Hearing Disorders*, *44*,(3), 350–353.

Helm-Estabrooks, N. (1986). Diagnosis and management of neurogenic stuttering in adults (pp. 198–217). In K. St. Louis (Ed.), *The atypical stutterer*. Orlando, FL: Academic Press.

Kent, R.D., & LaPointe, L.L. (1982). Acoustic properties of pathologic reiterative utterances: A case study of palilalia. *Journal of Speech and Hearing Research*, *25*, 95–99.

LaPointe, L.L., & Horner, J. (1981). Palilalia: A descriptive study of pathologic reiterative utterances. *Journal of Speech and Hearing Disorders*, *46*, 34–38.

Porch, B.E. (1967). *The Porch index of communicative ability*. Palo Alto, CA: Consulting Psychologists Press.

Schuell, H. (1965). *The Minnesota test for differential diagnosis of aphasia*. Minneapolis: University of Minnesota Press.

Yorkston, K., Beukelman, D., & Bell, K. (1988). *Clinical management of dysarthric speakers*. San Diego: College-Hill Press/Little, Brown.

SECTION II

UNUSUAL BEHAVIORS
ASSOCIATED WITH
HEAD INJURY

CHAPTER 4

MICHAEL COLLINS

██████████████████

TWENTY-SIX YEAR OLD WITH POST-TRAUMATIC ENCEPHALOPATHY

*T*he title of this book suggests that some diagnoses are more difficult than others. Certainly some are more perplexing than others. As this case history will demonstrate, however, their resolution may sometimes have less to do with our expertise than with a willingness to test traditional clinical wisdom, and to capitalize on our extensive literature and the experience of our peers.

PATIENT HISTORY

Our patient was a 26-year-old man with a complicated medical and psychiatric history, admitted for the assessment of his rehabilitation potential and for the evaluation of seizures. His parents reported that he had been dyslexic throughout his childhood, and had attempted suicide at least twice. Those attempts resulted in a two-year psychiatric hospitalization when he was 17. During that hospitalization, he attended high school and graduated when he was 19.

He spent the next several years in a variety of unskilled jobs. At the urging of his parents, he enlisted in the Air Force when he was 23. Soon after he had completed basic training, he was involved in a motor vehicle accident that reportedly resulted in a head injury and mild compression fracture of the sixth cervical vertebra. He later developed what were described as generalized seizures and memory deficits. He returned to his parents' home to recover. They reported that his behavior was normal, and that they did not notice any personality or behavioral changes. Approximately four months after the accident, when he had returned to active duty, he was charged with theft and passing bad checks. Over the next six months he became progressively more hostile, and reported being unable to recall events prior to the accident. Neuropsychological testing approximately ten months post-onset revealed a severe memory deficit and an IQ of 74, which represented a decline of 1.5 standard deviations from previous testing. The final diagnostic impression was of severe dementia, affecting left hemisphere functions more than right. Subsequently, his behaviors have been attributed to dementia, organic brain syndrome, post-traumatic encephalopathy, dementia secondary to trauma, and seizure disorder.

Since that time, numerous reports of violent acting out, nightmares, and episodic alcohol abuse have been noted. One year after the accident he was seen in an emergency room for what was reported to be a generalized tonoclonic seizure. He was treated with Dilantin. He reported one to two seizures per week, accompanied by severe frontal headaches. Physical examination at that time was normal. Our service received a request to evaluate a "26-year-old man with post-traumatic encephalopathy."

NEUROLOGICAL EXAMINATION

The neurologist found that cranial nerves III–XII were intact. Sensation was normal to light touch in vibration and pinprick tests, and motor strength was rated 4/5 for right grip and hand muscles, and 5/5 in all other groups. Reflexes were symmetric, including Romberg. Rapid hand motion and gait were normal. He was alert but irritable, and eye contact was poor. He denied depression or anxiety related to memory loss, and his thought content and form seemed intact. He was oriented to person, place, and time, and he remembered three of three objects after five minutes. He was unable to do serial sevens or proverbs, but his judgment and insight were judged to be "good." Laboratory testing yielded a normal urinalysis, white blood count, hematocrit, electrolytes, blood urea nitrogen, and creatinine. His Dilantin level of 2.3 mcg/ml was judged to be subtherapeutic.

One day after admission, he was observed to have what was described as a 30- to 60-second tonoclonic seizure, after which he was somnolent for approximately one hour. He was treated with Tegretol, and his Dilantin was gradually tapered.

During that admission, an MRI, CT scan, and EEG were performed. None showed any evidence of abnormality. These results agreed with those obtained during his initial hospitalization.

SPEECH AND LANGUAGE EVALUATION

AUDITORY COMPREHENSION AND RETENTION

During our initial interview, we noted no obvious functional deficits in auditory comprehension or retention. On the two primary auditory subtests of the Porch Index of Communicative Ability (PICA) (Porch, 1967), however, he required two repetitions, and nine of his responses were significantly delayed. Although he complained of profound memory deficits, and claimed to be unable to recall any significant events prior to his accident, he quickly recalled the topics of several conversations over a period of three days. Questions about events and locations he experienced after his accident were met with "I can't remember" or some variant.

READING

The patient's reported history of dyslexia made the interpretation of reading results difficult. On the two reading subtests of the PICA, he made only one incorrect response. Although the other 19 responses were correct, they were consistently incomplete and delayed.

WRITING

Writing, performed with his preferred right hand, was legible and well-formed, and oriented normally on the page. Spelling, grammar, and syntax, however, were remarkable. Responses such as, "Yous draw with pensil," and, "Yous opens door withs key," were typical. Pronouns were consistently misspelled, and "s" was added inappropriately to 28 of 46 words in his responses to subtest A. Grammar and syntax were generally adequate. A sample of his writing is shown in Figure 4-1.

MOTOR SPEECH

Range, velocity, and direction of movement of the functional components for speech were well within normal limits. Phrase length was within normal limits, but duration of phonation was significantly reduced; fundamental frequency and F_0 range were within normal limits; loudness and loudness change were normal; resonance was normal; and diadochokinetic rate was normal. Strength of jaw, lips, and tongue was normal, and all structures were symmetrical.

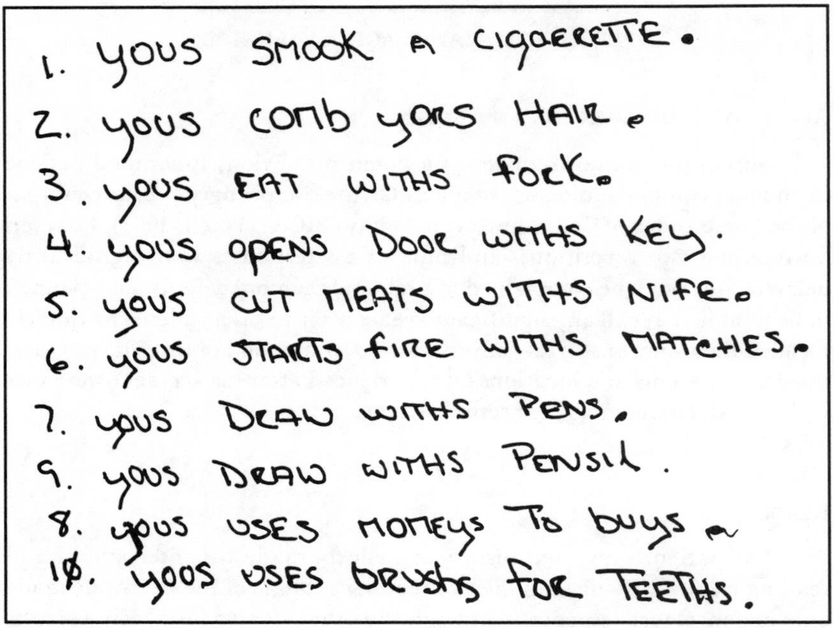

1. yous smook a cigaerette.
2. yous comb yors hair.
3. yous eat withs fock.
4. yous opens door withs key.
5. yous cut meats withs nife.
6. yous starts fire withs matches.
7. yous draw withs pens.
9. yous draw withs pensil.
8. yous uses moneys to buys a
10. yoos uses brushs for teeths.

Figure 4-1. PICA subtest A.

VERBAL PERFORMANCE

Superficially, our patient's speech was an amalgamation of diverse symptoms. Grammar and syntax were strikingly immature forms of their adult counterparts; for example, "Me write again?" and, "No can count past five." Despite the integrity of his speech systems and their functional components, he frequently sounded dysarthric. Although he was unable to sustain phonation beyond a few seconds on request, he usually spoke in sentences of normal duration. Prosody was frequently monotonous, but periods of normal prosody were equally frequent. Consonants, and sometimes vowels, were often misarticulated. In addition to these confusing symptoms, he was often nonfluent. This nonfluency was characterized predominately by pauses, prolongation of syllables, and repetition and revision of initial syllables. None of these nonfluencies was accompanied by secondary features.

He produced 36 words beginning with S, T, P, and C on the Word Fluency Measure (Borkowski, Benton, & Spreen, 1967), which was below the tenth decile for men his age but just within the normal range. Forty-three of his responses to the Boston Naming Test (Kaplan, Goodglass, & Weintraub, 1983) were correct. That performance was below the mean of 55.73 for normal adults with 12 years or less of education, but just within the normal range of 42 to 59. Vocabulary in conversation was intermittently sophisticated, and suggested a facility with language that he did not typically display.

We administered the PICA as a general measure of his communicative ability. His overall performance was at the seventy-second percentile for patients with left hemisphere lesions. Mean variability was 12.4. Performance by modality ranged from the thirty-fifth (auditory) to the ninety-ninth (visual and copying) percentiles. There was little variability across subtests, a rejection of one item on the simpler reading subtest (all other reading responses were correct), and dissimilar performance on the two most difficult subtests, I and A. Interestingly, none of his responses were distorted on subtest I, but of the 30 remaining verbal responses, 11 were distorted. Of those 30, only three were distorted similarly.

IMPRESSIONS

At this point, our formal test data had not contributed much to our diagnosis. Performance ranged from normal to disordered, but the pattern of those objective scores did not permit labeling. We had formed a subjective impression, but could not substantiate it. Our impression was based more on what we thought the patient was not than what we thought he was.

We did not believe that our patient's constellation of speech and language symptoms suggested an organic etiology. The primary feature of his spoken language, immature grammatical and syntactical forms, was not suggestive of an acquired aphasia. Aphasia is not a regression phenomenon in which the rules for adult discourse are somehow lost. Linguistic competence is relatively preserved in aphasic patients, despite their diminished performance. Perhaps because that is true, aphasic patients try very hard, and because language is so difficult for them the effort is obvious. This was not the case with our patient. When the effort was obvious, it was usually inappropriate.

We did not think that our patient was dysarthric. Dysarthria implies diminished control over the functional components of speech. His control was within normal limits for both speech and nonspeech tasks. Dysarthria is also characterized by relatively consistent errors; our patient's errors were inconsistent across sounds, stimuli, and situations.

We also did not feel that our patient was demented. His attention, relevance, frequent linguistic and cognitive sophistication, and appropriateness did not suggest a dementia.

In summary, we believed the probability was high that our patient was not aphasic, demented, or dysarthric. We also were certain that his behavioral profile was, at least to us, unique. By this time, however, we had nearly exhausted our measurement repertoire. It seemed we had only our clinical impressions to guide us as we left the familiar confines of our tests and our data base.

When we sought support in the literature, we found that Porch, Friden, and Porec (1977) had reported on their attempts to differentiate between aphasic patients and patients with a nonorganic component to their symptoms. In their study, aphasic patients and students feigning aphasia were given the PICA. From those test scores, discriminant functions were generated to classify those two groups of patients. They found the equation could differentiate these patients with a probability of .75.

To apply the equation to our patient's PICA scores, we first calculated subtest means. Fourteen of these subtests means were then multiplied by the weights generated by Porch and colleagues. These products were summed, and then added to a constant of +0.10615. The result was a score of +0.17485. According to Porch and his colleagues, scores of less than -0.279 are consistent with a diagnosis of nonaphasic (nonorganic) deficit. We now had some objective data to go with our subjective impressions.

THE ANSWER

In general terms, we thought that our patient's disorder was functional or affective. What gave rise to, and perpetuated, these symptoms was much less clear. Nevertheless, we felt that many of his symptoms were feigned. To our knowledge, this constellation of symptoms has not been described in association with central nervous system pathology. One of the most striking discrepancies displayed by our patient was between writing and speaking. He often spoke awkwardly and telegraphically, with no paraphasias, but wrote in more or less complete sentences with numerous paraphasias. No less striking was the intermittent presence of dysarthria. Usually, dysarthric speakers are almost the epitome of consistency, because their systems permit little variation in production. Aphasic, demented, and confused patients do not produce these errors either, unless they have more than one lesion. Finally, it was apparent that our patient was always able to communicate what he *wanted* to communicate.

To summarize, our impressions were influenced most strongly by the following:

1. Speech inconsistently dysarthric and not compatible with his normal functional components.
2. Written and spoken language more suggestive of a developmental disorder rather than an acquired disorder.
3. Atypical discrepancy between written and spoken language.

4. An extremely delayed development of symptoms.
5. Normal EEG, CT scan, and MRI on two occasions.
6. Performance on the PICA suggestive of a nonorganic component.
7. Reports by family and friends that his speech did not change until nearly two years following his accident.
8. Letters from the patient to his family written long after his accident revealed no significant deficits.

We were, of course, not completely certain of our diagnosis, nor had we ruled out the possibility of an organic component. Nine days after our evaluation, however, we were buoyed by the neuropsychological summary. The report concluded, "it is certainly unreasonable to accept his present scores as valid or reliable estimates of his actual ability levels." This opinion was based on the fact that he made reading errors on simple words and had no difficulty in identifying much more demanding words in the reading list; and that dense and protracted retrograde amnesia is a relatively rare finding in organically based amnestic syndromes. In addition, the appearance of significant memory complaint, of whatever description, some four months after the original injury, is extraordinary. The neuropsychologist was confident that a significant element of malingering and deliberate simulation of impairment contaminated the present neuropsychological profile. He did not exclude the possibility that the patient had bona fide post-traumatic encephalopathy, "albeit of a much lesser degree than what would be suggested by uncritical acceptance of his formal test scores."

CONCLUSION

We were perplexed by a disorder that was unique to us, and one for which we had no definitive, scientifically validated test. Fortunately, we were the beneficiaries of the experience of our colleagues as reflected in the literature available to us. We in turn share this unusual case, which we hope contributes to the literature relevant to such diagnostic dilemmas and ultimately to improved science-based tests.

REFERENCES

Borkowski, J.G., Benton, A.L., & Spreen, O. (1967). Word fluency and brain damage. *Neuropsychologia, 9*, 75–79.

Kaplan, E., Goodglass, H., & Weintraub, S. (1983). *Boston Naming Test*. Philadelphia: Lea and Febiger.

Porch, B. (1967). *The Porch Index of Communicative Ability.* Palo Alto, CA: Consulting Psychologists Press.

Porch, B., Friden, T., & Porec, J. (February 1977). *Objective differentiation of aphasic versus nonorganic patients.* Paper presented to the annual meeting of the International Neuropsychology Association, Santa Fe, New Mexico.

CHAPTER 5

BRENDA B. ADAMOVICH

BEHAVIORAL DISTURBANCES SECONDARY TO CLOSED HEAD INJURY AND MENTAL ILLNESSES

A woman (Mrs. A.) was referred for speech, language, and cognitive evaluations following a closed head injury. She exhibited several behaviors typically associated with closed head injury, including amnesia, hyperactivity, egocentricity, hypersexuality, confabulation, impaired social judgment, denial of illness, and confusion. This woman differed from other patients, however, with regard to the large number of behaviors evinced, the magnitude of her responses in each area, and a tendency to lose contact with reality. Our challenge was to gather the data necessary to substantiate these impressions, and to determine the etiology of the behavioral problems, in order to establish a successful rehabilitation program.

BRIEF HISTORY OF CASE

Mrs. A. was 34 years old when she sustained a severe closed head injury after the automobile she was driving was struck from behind by a drunk driver. She sustained left frontal cerebral focal lesions with diffuse brain damage and was admitted to the acute care hospital in December, 1982. Mrs. A. was in a coma for approximately 24 hours, and she experienced anterograde and retrograde post-traumatic amnesia. She had no recall of occurrences during the week following her accident. It has been suggested that post-traumatic amnesia for this length of time is indicative of severe injury (Karlsbeek, McLaurin, Harris, & Miller, 1980; Russell, 1932). This did not hold true in Mrs. A.'s case, however, as she eventually recovered to the point where she was ambulatory and evinced only mild cognitive and physical disabilities with mild right-sided weakness. Prior to her accident, Mrs. A. worked as a self-trained computer programming assistant with a major computer company. The mother of a 17-year-old son and 14-year-old daughter, she was an extremely intelligent, high school graduate with one year of college. According to both Mrs. A. and her husband, their marriage was sound and mutually supportive.

ASSESSMENT

Initial speech-language-cognition testing occurred two and a half weeks after her hospital admission. Diagnostic tests administered included portions of the Boston Diagnostic Aphasia Examination (BDAE) (Goodglass & Kaplan, 1983), the Detroit Tests of Learning Aptitude (DTLA) (Baker & Leland, 1959), the Minnesota Test of Differential Diagnosis of Aphasia (MTDDA) (Schuell, 1972), the Clinical Evaluation of Language Functions (CELF) (Semel & Wiig, 1980), the Boston Naming Test (BNT) (Kaplan, Goodglass, & Weintraub, 1983), the Reading Comprehension Battery for Aphasia (RCBA) (LaPointe & Horner, 1979), the Borkowski, Benton, and Spreen Word Fluency Task (Spreen & Benton, 1969), and nonstandardized assessments of immediate, short-term, and recent memory, attention to a selected task, linguistic organization abilities, and task-specific insight.

Mrs. A. was unable to provide the names or ages of her children. She followed only one-step commands with motoric perseveration; produced fluent, perseverative and neologistic speech with an inability to name common objects; exhibited poor sentence and paragraph comprehension; showed impaired memory and cognition (discrimination, organization, and reasoning). Many of her verbal responses were somewhat bizarre (see Table 5-1).

Mrs. A. made good cognitive and physical recovery during the first few weeks after her injury. At this time she had mild to moderate right-sided weakness and required minimal assistance with ambulation. As her cognitive abilities improved, the number of apparent bizarre behaviors increased along with a compulsive need to perform perfectly. Further questioning of the patient's husband revealed that Mrs. A. had a previous history of severe depression and general frustration, which was thought to be due to unmet

TABLE 5-1.
Examples of Mrs. A.'s bizarre verbal responses.*

Probe	Response
Describe how morning and afternoon are alike and different.	"Basically, the things that go on are in the same quality of what we carry."
Use the word *car* in a sentence.	"It means get out oven."
Use the word *carry* in a sentence.	"I can't use this word *carry* without a full deck."
All attempts at general conversation.	"Who are you? Why are you doing this?"

*These responses given during initial testing 2.5 weeks after her injury.

goals in her life. She had participated in several years of psychotherapy, and was in therapy at the time of her accident. Her emotional disturbance appeared to have been exacerbated by the head injury.

In addition to the assessment of cognitive and information processing deficits secondary to the head injury, extended behavioral assessments were indicated. Differential diagnostic considerations regarding the etiology of Mrs. A.'s behavioral disorders included: attentional disturbances, a frontal lobe syndrome, mental illness, and normal reactions to stress. When Mrs. A.'s extreme behavioral disturbances initially occurred (including agitation and physical abusiveness), attempts were made to control her behaviors through the use of Haldol. It should be noted that the use of drugs to control behaviors following head injury is the last method of choice because of their detrimental effect on information processing. It was subsequently decided that because Mrs. A.'s aggressive outbursts were not constant and she did not appear to be in danger of harming herself or others, the Haldol medication should be discontinued. Behavioral techniques then were initiated in an attempt to control her inappropriate behaviors.

ATTENTION

A variety of behaviors occur as a result of global disorders of attention or confusional states secondary to closed head injury (Geschwind, 1982). The behaviors are summarized in Table 5-2. The behaviors not exhibited by Mrs. A. are identified by asterisks.

Loss of coherence refers to an abrupt shifting of topics of discussion or actions. Mrs. A. frequently displayed this behavior making it difficult to converse or interact with her.

Paramnesias refer to a distortion rather than a loss of memory. Although

TABLE 5-2.
Behaviors characteristic of global attentional
disorders (confusional states) secondary to closed
head injury.

Loss of coherence
Paramnesia
Error propagation
*Occupational jargon
Inattention to environmental stimuli
*Isolated or predominant writing disturbance
Unconcern or denial of illness
Playful behavior

Adapted from Geschwind, 1982.
*Behaviors not exhibited by Mrs. A.

answers are essentially incorrect, elements of the correct answer are present, thus suggesting that some aspect of the information has been learned. Mrs. A. knew she was not at home, but thought that she was in a jail, not a hospital.

Error propagation refers to the tendency to bring other items in the environment into apparent coherence with an error that has already been made. Because Mrs. A. believed she was in a jail, error propagation resulted in her determination that the nurses and other hospital personnel were guards.

Inattention to environmental stimuli refers to a failure to use environmental information during the formulation of a response or conclusion. For example, Mrs. A. did not attend to environmental cues such as the absence of bars on the windows and locks on the doors when she insisted that she was in jail.

Mrs. A. showed very little concern regarding her present state or future plans. She denied cognitive deficits and blamed others for her errors.

FRONTAL LOBE SYNDROME

Common focal brain lesions secondary to direct impact closed head injury are seen in frontopolar, orbitofrontal, and anterior temporal areas. Behaviors that typically result from frontal lobe damage, as well as those behaviors evidenced by Mrs. A., are summarized in Table 5-3.

Mrs. A. was grandiose in her actions, manner of speaking, and her assumptions. She paraded about in a rather queenly way and seemed to "look down her nose" at others as she spoke in a proper, superior manner. She was convinced that the company where she had worked prior to her accident would be forced to close in her absence. Even her neologistic talk

TABLE 5-3.
Behaviors characteristic of frontal lobe disturbances.

Cortical overresponsiveness	Lack of concern for present and
Fantastical, grandiose associations	future
Pressured speech	Decreased initiative
*Tangential speech	Decreased attention
Disturbance of time sense	Decreased memory (episodic and
Gap filling	everyday)
Decreased information regulation	Gross disinhibition
and integration	Loss of impulse control
Delusional denial of illness	Erotic behavior
Emotional lability	Sexual exhibitionism
Alterations in personality	Lewd remarks
(childishness, egoism, irritability)	Confabulation (right frontal: more
Euphoria alternating with depression	frequent)

Adapted from Hecaen and Albert, 1978; Joseph, 1986.
*Behavior not exhibited by Mrs. A.

was presented in an extremely sophisticated, grandiose manner. Her pressured speech was delivered with an excited emotional tone, although she conversed rather easily. Emotional lability ranged from periods of extreme rage to episodes of uncontrollable crying. She displayed an irritability that often resulted in loss of control with no warning in response to petty situations. In her husband's presence, Mrs. A. behaved in a childish manner. She expected a protective, father-like response, and became angry if her husband did not comply. Both the family and the rehabilitation team found it difficult to deal effectively with her gross disinhibition, loss of impulse control, erotic behavior, sexual exhibitionism, and lewd remarks. Mrs. A.'s husband was extremely concerned following a weekend leave of absence from the hospital during which time Mrs. A. wanted to spend the entire weekend in their bedroom having sexual relations with total disregard for their two teenage children who were also in the home. Masturbation and inappropriate sexual comments were frequent occurrences. When asked by an elderly female hospital volunteer how she was doing, she responded, "I'm horny as hell. How about you?" On another occasion, she grabbed the behind of a young male aide and commented, "Doesn't he have a great ass?"

NORMAL COPING REACTION

As the human brain attempts to integrate and again make sense of perceptions of the world following closed head trauma, dysfunctions of perception and integration may result in distorted conclusions, leading to distress and confusion (Barry, 1986). An adjustment disorder secondary to maladaptive reactions to stress generally occurs within three months of the onset of an identifiable stressor (Williams, 1980). Adjustment disorders are characterized by behaviors that are similar to, but far exceed, normal and expectable reactions to the stressor. Once irritated, Mrs. A. would often become outraged, and physically aggressive. While at home on a leave of absence, she threw an iron at her children and tore down all of the kitchen curtains.

MENTAL DISORDERS

According to Fahy, Irving, and Millac (1967), 17 of 22 patients studied with severe head injury evinced psychiatric sequelae. These disorders include neuroses or exaggeration of normal reactions, and psychoses in which severe disruptions of thought processing occur. A psychotic individual is illogical and appears to have lost contact with reality.

NEUROSES

Behaviors characteristic of neuroses are summarized in Table 5-4. Those behaviors not evinced by Mrs. A. are indicated by asterisks. Post-traumatic stress disorders are characterized by recognizable stressors, a tendency to re-experience the trauma or accident, decreased responsiveness or involvement in the external world, hyperalertness, and a sleep disturbance. Mrs. A. evinced all of these behaviors with the exception of decreased responsiveness/involvement in the external world.

The behavioral characteristics of an organic personality syndrome secondary to head trauma are also presented in Table 5-4. Mrs. A. evinced all of these behaviors. A marked apathy or indifference was evident during treatment sessions even though attempts were continually made to relate treatment goals to relevant functional activities. She did not seem to be concerned about resuming a normal life, and would not participate in any discussions regarding specific goals, including returning home, returning to work, or getting involved in the activities of her children.

Behaviors characterizing secondary mania following head trauma are also presented in Table 5-4. Generally, people with this disorder have no history of previous psychiatric illness, but, as noted earlier, Mrs. A. had undergone psychotherapy for several years prior to her injury. Secondary mania following head trauma in 20 patients has been described by Shukla and colleagues (1987). These investigators suggested that predisposing factors included post-traumatic amnesia and post-traumatic seizures.

TABLE 5-4.
Behaviors characteristic of neuroses.

Post-traumatic Stress Disorder
Recognizable stressor
Reexperiences trauma
*Decreased responsiveness/involvement in external world
Hyperalertness
Sleep disturbances

Secondary Mania Due to Head Trauma
*Absence of previous psychiatric illness
Negative family history for bipolar illness
Close temporal proximity of head trauma to subsequent
mania:
● Hyperactivity
● Push of speech
● Grandiosity
● Flight of ideas
● Decreased sleep
● Distractibility
● Lack of judgment

Organic Personality Syndrome Secondary to Head Trauma
Mood swings: Lability, explosive temper outbursts, sudden
crying
Decreased impulse control: Poor social judgment, sexual
indiscretions, etc.
Marked apathy or indifference
Suspiciousness or paranoid ideation
Denial
Childishness
Grief
Anger
Depression
Decreased self-image
Decreased self-esteem

Phobic Neurosis
*Irrational, displaced fears of objects or situations (e.g.,
dirt, bacteria, cancer, crowds)
*Morbid anxiety
*Avoidance of feared object or situation

Anxiety Neurosis
  *Persistent feeling of dread, apprehension and impending
    disaster not referable to specific objects or events
  *Disturbances of physiological functions: Generalized
    visceral tension, hyperventilation, cardiac and pyloric
    spasms, intestinal irritability, diarrhea or constipation,
    palpitation, tachycardia, respiratory distress, etc.
  *Fainting, weakness, nausea, tremor and perspiration of
    hands and face
  *Depression
  *Sleeplessness
  *Irritability
  *Restlessness
  *Outbursts of aggressiveness
  *Chronic fatigue

Hysterical Neurosis
  *Amnesia
  *Dissociative delirium
  *Hallucinations

Hypochondria
  *Obsessive preoccupation and concern about health
    and organs

Obsessive Compulsive Neurosis
  *Thoughts persistently thrust into consciousness against
    conscious desire
  *Persistently repeats unreasonable thoughts and acts
    uncontrollably
  *Punctilious, rigid, fastidious, formal and meticulous
  Lacks capacity for relaxation
  *Tendency toward literal obedience
  *Exaggerated sense of duty,
  *Cannot make decisions
  *Daydreaming, introverted, self-centered

Conversion Reaction
  *Anxiety converted into functional symptoms in organs or
    parts of the body innervated by the sensorimotor
    nervous system

Depression Neurosis
  *Self-deprecating behavior
  *Crying

Adapted from Bond, 1979; Kolb, 1977; Levin, Grossman, & Kelly, 1979; Williams, 1980.
*Behaviors not exhibited by Mrs. A.

PSYCHOSES

Psychotic disturbances include paranoid reactions, schizophrenic reactions, or disorders of thought and affective reactions, or disorders of emotion (Williams, 1980). Behaviors that characterize paranoid psychoses are summarized in Table 5-5. Mrs. A. evinced all but one of these behaviors. As indicated in Table 5-5, psychotic patients reportedly experience "intricate delusions with an otherwise intact personality." Mrs. A. did evince delusions, but she also exhibited many other personality disturbances, including hallucinations, bizarre delusions, and incoherence.

Mrs. A. mistrusted everyone. She was found on several occasions with packed suitcases in the elevator "attempting to escape from prison." She was convinced that the therapists and nurses were gathering legal information against her by keeping track of her correct and incorrect responses in therapy sessions and on the nursing unit. Although her husband was quite devoted and seldom missed a day of visiting with her, Mrs. A. was convinced that he was having an affair and would become hysterical if he were even five minutes late for visiting hours. A cold and unemotional affect was observed with regard to her two children. When questioned regarding their preparations for the beginning of the school year, she showed no concern and no interest in pursuing the discussion. When the children were in her presence, she usually would ignore them and pay no attention to any personal needs or concerns they expressed.

SCHIZOPHRENIC PSYCHOSES: DISORDERS OF THOUGHT

Mrs. A. also was extremely manipulative. Her intelligence allowed her to devise elaborate, believable stories to support her point of view. When her frustration increased due to failure at clinical tasks, Mrs. A. convinced her husband that she should discontinue therapy due to an unresolvable personality clash between the therapist and herself.

Behaviors characterizing schizophrenic psychoses are summarized in Table 5-5, as well as the behaviors displayed by Mrs. A. Delusions refer to false personal beliefs based on incorrect inferences about external reality, which are firmly held despite evidence to the contrary. Specific types of delusions include persecution, control, grandeur, jealousy, and reference (Williams, 1980). Several examples of delusions have been discussed previously. Mrs. A., for example, felt that she was gaining weight, when in fact she was actually losing weight. To deal with her belief she began to compulsively exercise. An exercise mat was put into her room to prevent injuries as the nurses would continually find her vigorously exercising, even in the middle of the night.

Head injured patients commonly evince paramnesias or the distortion of memory, resulting in incorrect answers with elements of the correct answer

TABLE 5-5.
Behavioral characteristics of psychoses.

Paranoid Psychoses	Schizophrenic Psychoses: Disorders of Thought	Affective Psychoses: Disorders of Emotion
Mistrust of people: • Guarded • Avoid accepting warranted blame • Search for confirmation of biases Hypersensitive: • "Makes mountains out of molehills" • Readiness to counterattack • Inability to relax Restricted affectivity Appears cold and unemotional Logical, highly systematized *Intricate delusions with personality otherwise intact	Bizarre delusions Hallucinations: • In presence of clear consciousness • Auditory (most common) Incoherence Poverty of content speech Flat or inappropriate affect Grossly disorganized behavior Ambivalence (blending of love and hate) Negativism Anxiety Emotional withdrawal Use of neologisms	Extreme fluctuations of mood: Manic/depressed Disturbance in behavior: Depression, fearfulness, anxiety, unreliability, phobias, panic, suspiciousness, anger, etc. Delusions of persecution Hallucinations Disturbance in thought: Attention, concentration, memory and abstract thinking Impaired empathetic response Rigidity of thought process

Adapted from Carberry & Burd, 1986; Carlson & Goodwin, 1973; Kolb, 1977; Williams, 1980.
*Behaviors not exhibited by Mrs. A.

present. One example is reduplicative paramnesia, in which certain items are duplicated, so that the hospital may be regarded as a school and the therapists as teachers (Geschwind, 1982). Paramnesias differ from delusions in that they represent an attempt to use past experience to bring order to the world in the midst of much confusion. For example, most young patients have little experience with hospitals and more experience with schools, so it is logical for them to imagine that the hospital is a school.

Hallucinations refer to false auditory, gustatory, visual, and haptic sensory perceptions. Hallucinations indicate psychotic disturbances if they coexist with gross impairments in reality testing (Williams, 1980). Mrs. A. experienced auditory hallucinations. She frequently asked people to be quiet as she was "trying to hear what was being said to her." She would then appear to be struggling to attend to information. She would not respond when asked who was speaking to her. She frequently reported the sensation of terrible taste in her mouth.

Mrs. A. experienced gustatory, visual, and haptic hallucinations. On one occasion she asked for a cigarette. When I responded that I did not smoke and I did not have a cigarette, she strongly persisted, claiming, "You do have a cigarette. There's one right in your pocket." When given the opportunity to examine the contents of my pocket, she pulled out an imaginary cigarette, thanked me, lit the cigarette with an imaginary match, and began to smoke the cigarette. On another occasion, Mrs. A. offered me a piece of candy from an imaginary box of candy. She became extremely agitated when I explained that I did not see any candy. She began to eat the imaginary pieces of candy and replied, "It's just as well you don't want any because there's more candy for me."

AFFECTIVE REACTION (DISORDERS OF EMOTION)

Behaviors characterizing affective psychoses are also summarized in Table 5-5. Mrs. A. evinced all of these behaviors. Her mood swings ranged in a relatively short period of time from very jovial, happy manic states to states of rage followed by depression. Impaired empathic responses were apparent as Mrs. A. was not sensitive at all to the feelings of those around her, including her own children and husband. She was extremely egocentric and showed concern only for her own feelings and well-being.

The cause of the thought disturbances (including concentration, memory, and problem solving) was unclear; these disturbances can occur as a result of affective psychoses or secondary to closed head injury.

DISCUSSION AND CONCLUSION

Mrs. A. evinced many cognitive disorders and behavioral problems. It was difficult to determine whether these disorders were secondary to (1) her head injury, or to (2) psychiatric disturbances that occurred secondary to her head injury, or that were previously present and were exacerbated by the head injury. The etiology of the behavioral deficits was considered to be an important variable in the establishment of the treatment plan. Attempts were made to work with a psychologist who had treated Mrs. A. prior to her accident in an attempt to gain insight into the etiology dilemma. Unfortunately, although this person understood psychiatric disturbances, he lacked an understanding of the behaviors that occur secondary to closed head injury. For example, he was not aware of the severe memory disturbances which typically occur following head trauma. When asked to review his findings at a team conference, he reported a psychotic disturbance based on the fact that Mrs. A. denied participation in lengthy counseling sessions which has occurred less than 24 hours earlier.

The results of the diagnostic assessment of Mrs. A. suggested the presence of attentional disturbances, cognitive disturbances, and information processing disturbances. Behavior problems appeared to be secondary to a frontal lobe syndrome, stress reactions, and mental illness. Neurotic tendencies prior to Mrs. A.'s accident were exacerbated following the head injury. Mrs. A. also had become psychotic following her accident, and psychiatric intervention was indicated. Rehabilitation programs designed to treat her attention, cognitive, and information processing deficits were severely limited by her neurotic and psychiatric behaviors. Participation in group therapy sessions was not appropriate as Mrs. A.'s bizarre behaviors would frighten the other group members and she would completely disrupt the group. For these reasons, it was recommended that rehabilitation treatment be temporarily discontinued until the patient was able to receive help for her psychiatric disorder. Unfortunately, the treatment of the psychiatric disorder was hindered by Mrs. A.'s cognitive problems, including poor attention, memory, and problem solving. A specialized program for psychiatrically disturbed, head injured patients would have been the most ideal placement for Mrs. A. Unfortunately, as is true in most areas of the country at this time, a program of this nature was not available.

REFERENCES

Baker, H. & Leland, B. (1959). *Detroit tests of learning aptitude* (revised). New York: Bobbs-Merrill Co.

Barry, P. (1986). A psychological perspective of acute brain injury rehabilitation. *Cognitive Rehabilitation, 4*(4), 18-21.

Bond, M.R. (1979). Stages of recovery from severe head injury with special references to late outcome. *Internation Rehabilitation Medicine, 1*, 155.

Carberry, H. & Burd, B. (1986). Individual psychotherapy with the brain injured adult. *Cognitive Rehabilitation, 4*(4), 22-25.

Carlson, G.A. & Goodwin, F.K. (1973). The stages of mania. *Archives of General Psychitary, 28*, 221-228.

Fahy, T.J., Irving, M.H., & Millac, P. (1967). Severe head injuries. *Lancet*, 751-754.

Geschwind, H. (1982). Disorders of attention: A frontier in neuropsychology. *Philosophical Transactions of the Royal Society of London, 298*, 173-185.

Goodglass, H. & Kaplan, E. (1983). *The assessment of aphasia and related disorders* (2nd ed.). Philadelphia: Lea and Febiger.

Hecaen, H. & Albert, M.L. (1978). *Human neuropsychology*. New York: John Wiley.

Joseph, R. (1986). Confabulation and delusional denial: Frontal lobe and lateralized influences. *Journal of Clinical Psychology, 42*(3), 507-520.

Kaplan, E., Goodglass, H., & Weintraub, S. (1983). *Boston naming test*. Philadelphia: Lea and Febiger.

Karlsbeek, W.D., McLaurin, R.L., Harris, B.S.H., III, & Miller, J.D. (1980). The national head and spinal cord injury survey: Major findings. *Journal of Neurosurgery, 53*, 519.

Kolb, L.C. (1977). *Modern clinical psychiatry*. Philadelphia: W.B. Saunders.

LaPointe, L. & Horner, J. (1979). *Reading comprehension battery for aphasia*. Tigard, OR: C.C. Publications.

Levin, H.S., Grossman, R.G., & Kelly, P.J. (1979). Aphasic disorder in patients with closed head injury. *Journal of Neurology, Neurosurgery, and Psychiatry, 50*, 412-422.

Russell, W.R. (1932). Cerebral involvement in head injury. *Brain, 55*, 549-603.

Schuell, H. (1972). *The Minnesota test for differential diagnosis of aphasia* (rev. ed.). Minneapolis: University of Minnesota Press.

Semel, E. & Wiig, E. (1980). *Clinical evaluation of language functions*. Columbus, OH: Charles Merrill.

Shukla, S., Cook, B.J., Mukherjee, S., Godwin, C., & Miller, M.G. (1987). Mania following head trauma. *American Journal of Psychiatry, 144*(1), 93-96.

Spreen, O. & Benton, A.L. (1969). *Neuro-sensory center comprehensive examination for aphasia*. Victoria, BC: University of Victoria, Neuropsychology Laboratory.

Williams, J.B.W. (Ed.). (1980). *Diagnostic and statistical manual of mental disorders* (3rd ed.). DSM-III Washington, DC: American Psychiatric Association.

SECTION III

PSYCHOGENIC VERSUS
ORGANIC ETIOLOGIES IN
PATIENTS WITH SEVERE
COMMUNICATION
PROBLEMS

CHAPTER 6

JON G. LYON

A CASE OF PROLONGED RESPONSE LATENCIES: PHYSIOLOGICAL OR PSYCHOLOGICAL ETIOLOGY?

*O*ur introduction to Mr. R. was a consult from general medicine that read:

> 67 yo w male with a one day history of questionable receptive and expressive aphasia vs depression with a slow response. TIAs or depression?

Our initial exposure to this patient three days post-onset led us not into the diagnostic quandary of aphasia vs. depression as anticipated from this consult. Rather we found ourselves struggling over two separate diagnostic dilemmas: (1) Was the disorder of physiological or psychological origin and (2) if physiological, where might one expect to locate the lesion? Ten days after the onset of this disorder, a computed tomograph (CT) definitively resolved these issues.

The case is presented here as a test of your clinical investigative skills; a sort of "who-done-it?" More specifically, its aim is to challenge your ability to sort through relevant facts, call upon your acquired clinical knowledge and intuition, and, ultimately, to render valid diagnosis and etiology. The data are chronologically ordered as they were observed and uncovered.

BRIEF HISTORY OF CASE

Mr. R., a 67-year-old retired truck driver, awoke before dawn on a June morning and proceeded to shower, shave, and dress. His wife, finding this behavior highly uncharacteristic, attempted to determine his motives for leaving the house so early. Mr. R., however, appeared not to understand any inquiry, nor did he initiate any conversational speech. Although slightly "dazed," he continued unerringly in his preparation to leave the house. He wandered out into the front yard, where he stood perfectly still for an extended period before uttering the word "Vets." Mrs. R. interpreted this to mean the VA Medical Center and immediately drove him to this facility.

Mr. R.'s recent medical history was significant because of a brief hospital admission six months earlier. At that time, the presenting symptoms included "burning eyes," loss of balance, and weakness in all four extremities. These symptoms recurred several times over a three-day period and lasted approximately 20 minutes. They were diagnosed as transient ischemic attacks, possibly linked to a history of chronic heart failure (open heart bypass surgery in 1979; angioplasty in 1985). There was no interruption in his ability to communicate during any of these transitory episodes. He was placed on an anticoagulant, monitored for a five-day duration, and discharged. His past medical history was not significant for any other chronic illnesses. He had no known documented history of psychoses or neuroses.

Mr. R. was a native American speaker, right-handed, and had completed eight years of formal education. He resided with his wife in their private home.

TESTING

THE NEUROLOGICAL EXAMINATION

One day post-onset, Mr. R.'s neurological findings were mildly brisk deep tendon reflexes for both upper and lower extremities on the left side of the body, and a left extensor plantar response. There was no muscular weakness or loss of sensation on either side, nor were any of the cranial nerves involved. Communication was reported as largely intact receptively, although expression was limited to a few written words and use of pantomime. Later in the neurological exam, Mr. R. was reported to have verbalized several single words. The most striking feature of his neurological exam, however, was a pronounced delay (10–15 seconds) between stimulus and any expressive act (gestural, graphic, or verbal).

THE SPEECH AND LANGUAGE EVALUATION

Three days post-onset, an initial speech–language evaluation was conducted. It consisted of an informal speech–language screening battery and portions of the Boston Diagnostic Aphasia Examination (BDAE) (Goodglass & Kaplan, 1983).

FIRST IMPRESSIONS

Mr. R. was alert and attentive and appeared fully oriented. We saw no traces of the mental confusion ascribed to him upon admission. His eye contact and responsiveness to the examiner was consistent and appropriate throughout the evaluation. There was no visible motor weakness of any extremity or articulator. He gestured appropriately when using hand, arm, or facial movements, although the initiation of these movements was reduced in number. Simply stated, with the exception of his difficulty participating in a verbal dialogue, he appeared to be a normal, healthy 67-year-old man.

SPEECH AND LANGUAGE TEST RESULTS

GENERAL TEST BEHAVIOR. Throughout the evaluation, Mr. R.'s cooperation and willingness to perform requested tasks was exemplary. He never appeared to purposefully withhold or delay any response, but took 5 to 12 seconds before he seemed able to initiate any response. When questioned about this behavior, Mr. R. reported that he immediately understood the nature of my requests, but that he could not get his mind "to work" for a short period; "It is as though it is stuck and then it pops out."

AUDITORY COMPREHENSION. Mr. R. accurately completed all sections of the auditory comprehension subtests from the BDAE, although with penalties for prolonged delays. He did experience two errors on the Complex Ideational subtest, but was able to self-correct one of these following his usual delay. More remarkable was the apparent difference in the latency of response between pointing (identifying pictured stimuli or body parts or following full sentence commands) and verbalization (answering "yes" or "no" to questions). When asked to point to pictures, his latency was, on the average, 3 or 4 seconds less than when asked to verbally answer yes/no questions. Yet when the examiner requested that yes/no questions be answered solely with a head nod, delays were commensurate with verbal responses. Repeated efforts to get him to respond "as quickly as possible" resulted in no measurable change in response latency. Also, no difference in latency occurred when it was announced that the same question would be repeated over consecutive trials.

READING COMPREHENSION. Reading was good for sentence completion tasks and short paragraph comprehension. Longer, more abstract stimuli were not tested at this time. Printed simple or complex commands were carried out unerringly, although, as before, with significant delays. As with auditory comprehension, printed instructions which required him to point to objects within the room or to body parts appeared to elicit quicker responses than written stimuli requiring a verbal response (reading aloud).

CONVERSATIONAL SPEECH. Conversational speech was noticeably reduced in phrase length, although grammatical form was preserved. Content was intact. Again, pronounced delays preceded all responses. On occasion, delays occurred within longer utterances (4–8 words). There was no dysarthric quality to his speech. There was a reduction in vocal loudness (hypophonia) which was noted by Mr. R. and his wife from the time of onset.

NAMING. Confrontation and responsive naming as measured from the BDAE was intact, again with an 8 to 12 second latency preceding each response. Less familiar, more abstract items from an informal naming probe (bifocals, eyelets of a shoe, a hinge on a pair of glasses) were identified accurately with no observable difference in response latency when compared to familiar, common objects. On a divergent naming task, Mr. R. recalled only five animals in one minute. However, when he was permitted to continue on for nearly six minutes with uninterrupted recall his total was 24. Also, responsive naming, although accurate, failed to shorten previous response latencies.

AUTOMATIC SPEECH. Counting and reciting the days of the week and letters of the alphabet resulted in delays of eight seconds between each item in the respective series. Efforts to accelerate that rate proved ineffective. Singing or recitation of familiar rhymes did not increase his rate of response either.

Significantly though, some elements of "automatic speech" were initiated without the standard 8 to 12 second delay. When we entered Mr. R.'s room, he responded to the question, "How are you?" with only a brief delay (1–3 seconds). Similarly, several minimally delayed, automatic replys were observed to familiar questions within the evaluation. When departing, he quickly responded with a "bye." However, when any of these automatic utterances were brought to a volitional level (Would you please say "bye"?), the response delays recurred.

VERBAL REPETITION. Single words, short phrases, and longer phrases were repeated accurately with the same eight-second initiation delays. Once initiated, single words and short phrases were repeated in their entirety without pause. On longer sentences, however, he would repeat "chunks" with 8 to 12 second delays between phrase groups.

Length of response was not the sole determiner of whether delays fell within verbal repetitions. When requested to continue repetition of "baseball," he responded without an eight-second delay between words. Yet, when given the instruction to repeat the word baseball twice, an eight-second delay did occur between these words. Possibly the second process required an additional cognitive operation, thus the need for an intervening delay.

Literal or verbal paraphasias were minimal or absent throughout the speech tasks. Occasionally, he indicated that he could not produce any response. Whether this was due to initiation problems or retrieval problems was unclear.

WRITTEN EXPRESSION. When asked to write out the names of objects within a room, Mr. R.'s responses were accurate but, again, noticeably delayed. On longer words he paused between letters and occasionally omitted or reversed letters. Short words were accurately written out at a normal pace once the initial delay had elapsed.

AUDIOLOGICAL TESTING

All audiological screening measures were within normal limits.

SUMMARY OF SPEECH AND LANGUAGE FINDINGS

Our initial evaluation of Mr. R. pointed to a relatively intact internal linguistic system. There were no marked deficits in auditory or reading comprehension, word retrieval, or written expression. In addition, there were minimal or no literal or verbal paraphasias present in his spoken language. There was no dysarthria, although vocal loudness was diminished. Unquestionably the most pronounced deficit was his inability to purposefully initiate any communicative action without significant delay. We noted no "groping" or "mispositioning" of limbs or articulators on highly skilled motoric tasks. Motoric expressions were simply delayed. Athough the delays varied according to the task involved, responses requiring pointing or gestured actions were more immediate than spoken responses. Only the most automatic responses elicited in a highly appropriate and predictable context were produced within normal limits. When these same utterances were brought to a conscious, volitional level, the 8 to 12 second latencies again were seen.

NEUROPSYCHOLOGICAL EVALUATION

Mr. R. was evaluated by our staff neuropsychologist in the first three days post-onset, and his primary finding of marked response delays echoed our own. He underscored the fact that Mr. R. had no known history of psychogenic problems. Furthermore, he noted that Mr. R.'s response delays were not uniform. He found some of Mr. R.'s responses to be immediate (e.g., to the command "close your eyes" and to the question: Are you getting tired?), while a majority were of a longer delay.

A neuropsychological mental status evaluation was administered six days post-onset. Test findings were described as "highly inconsistent," although basic cognitive abilities appeared to be "intact." When attempting to judge whether this disability was of a physiological or psychological origin, he concluded that there was "support for both positions." However, he did indicate that if the behavior were organically based, the frontal lobes may be involved.

PSYCHOLOGICAL EVALUATION

Two days after his neuropsychological evaluation, Mr. R. was seen by a staff psychologist to rule out the diagnosis of depression. The psychologist questioned Mr. R.'s comprehension of language at the time. However, he noted that his affect was "blunted, stable, and mildly intact." He also noted that Mr. R. did not relate well within their communique. Mr. R. did not report any feelings of depression. This professional's opinion was that Mr. R., indeed, had incurred a physiological event compatible with frontal lobe atrophy (easily fatigued; apparent lack of concern; pseudo-depression).

DISCUSSION

Did Mr. R. suffer a vascular insult, or was this a manifestation of a depressed mental state?

The data, even from the initial case history, suggested that the latter diagnosis was highly improbable. The onset had been sudden and unlinked to any known psychological or emotional strain. There was no history of any prior psychoses or neuroses, especially in terms of affect or mood changes. Also, recall that the staff psychologist found no supporting evidence for a depressive condition. Thus, although it was possible that the behaviors we observed were the result of depression, it was unlikely.

If not depression, then could there have been a hysterical conversion component to Mr. R.'s behavior, or were the symptoms observed solely the result of a vascular accident?

Solomon (1985) defines hysterical conversion as the presence of symptoms or signs that the patient erroneously believes to be of an organic origin.

Commonly the onset of this disorder is abrupt. This certainly conforms to the appearance of Mr. R.'s disorder. In addition, hysterical patients usually are bland and indifferent to their defect, characteristics attributed to Mr. R. by the staff psychologist. Also, symptoms from a hysterical conversion generally do not conform completely and consistently to any known organically based disorder. The "abnormal" clinical findings in Mr. R. were pronounced latency periods, slightly heightened deep tendon reflexes on the left side of the body, and a positive left Babinski sign. Such findings suggest pathology in the contralateral, right cerebral hemisphere. But Mr. R.'s inability to initiate or sustain speech was in direct contrast to the verbal impulsiveness and/or verbosity that Myers (1984, 1986) reports as characteristic of right hemisphere impaired patients. In addition, there was the variability in response latencies for different types of expressive modes (gestured vs. verbal), as well as certain automatic, less propositional interactions. Thus, his behavioral and neurological findings did not conform to our expectations. Solomon (1985) noted that most patients experiencing a hysterical conversion had a previous history of psychoses or neuroses dating back into their youth. As far as we knew, no evidence of such episodes existed in Mr. R.'s past.

If this was not a hysterical conversion disorder, what lesion location might account for Mr. R.'s major symptoms?

Luria (1966) speaks of a frontal dynamic aphasia (FDA) where internal language, grammatical form, and word retrieval are largely intact. He states, "the dominant symptom is difficulty in the ecphoria of the whole expression or a disturbance of 'speech initiative' " (p. 212). Yet in Mr. R.'s case, there was a lack of conformity to other features that Luria lists as representative for FDA. Seemingly, most patients with FDA repeat without any impairment in content or latency of response. In fact, Luria maintains that such patients often do relatively well in the use of familiar, short phrases. The difficulty arises when asked to expound a sequential list of elements from within a series. He reports that FDA patients often revert to echolalia of portions of the question asked. We did not sample Mr. R.'s ability to recount sequential tasks at the time of this evaluation, so he did not exhibit unimpaired repetition skills, nor could he produce more familiar phrases without prolonged response latencies.

Ardila and Lopez (1984) view Luria's FDA as one of two types of transcortical motor aphasia. A second form of transcortical motor aphasia is a result of a lesion in the supplementary motor area (SMA) of the left hemisphere. In contrasting the two forms, they maintain that a patient with an SMA lesion tries to communicate, but cannot initiate the necessary processes to do so. In contrast, the patient with FDA (e.g., a lesion just anterior to Broca's area) lacks the volition to even attempt to communicate. According to this differentiation, Mr. R. might be expected to have an SMA lesion.

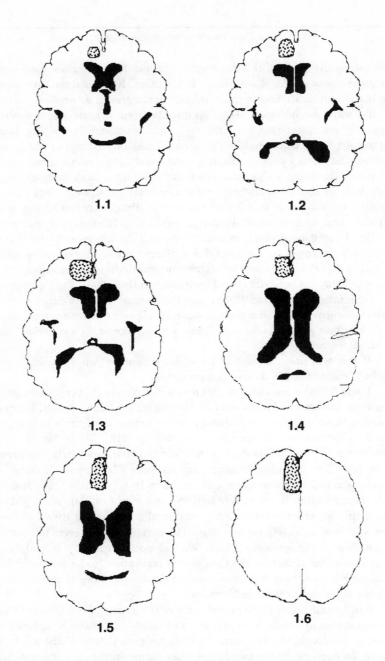

Figure 6-1. Templates from Mr. R.'s CT scan (ten days post-onset). Initial cut (1.1) at level of the third ventricle and subsequent cuts progressing rostrally until above the lateral ventricles (1.6).

But SMA patients also are described as having phonemic paraphasias during repetition without any significant delay in response latency. Also, SMA patients reportedly are unable to read letters within a word and exhibit marked deficits in writing due to slowness and paragraphias. None of these latter symptoms held true for Mr. R.

Finally, we reviewed the works of Damasio (1981), who reported on cases of mutism. Unlike aphasias, cortically based mutisms result in an absence or significant reduction in verbal output, although linguistic and cognitive skills are generally intact.

> Patients with mutism are aspontaneous both in relation to their non-existent speech as well as in relation to other motor behaviors, for example, gestural communication and motor drive toward new stimuli. However, if stimulated enough, they can repeat words and sentences normally, and their comprehension of aural and written language is intact. (p. 38)

Mr. R.'s verbal repetition was not normal because of aspontaneity. Even with repeated stimulation, this deficit remained. Damasio noted that acquired cortically based mutisms often result from lesions very high in the left frontal lobe above the lateral ventricle. Furthermore, they usually extend to the white matter along the mesial portion of the frontal lobe, adjacent to the medical longitudinal fissure.

In the end, our literature review uncovered no other case just like Mr. R. Despite his uniqueness, we leaned more to a neurological than psychological basis for this disorder. We concluded that if a lesion was present, it resided in the left frontal lobe approximate to the supplementary motor area (Ardila & Lopez, 1984; Damasio, 1981). Ten days post-onset, confirmation of a left frontal lesion was obtained from a CT scan (see Figure 6-1). Although the lesion was anterior to the supplementary motor area and along the mesial surface of the left frontal lobe, caudally its course was more extensive than anticipated, reaching a level of the third ventricle (Figure 6-1.1). There was no evidence from the CT scan of right hemisphere pathology that could account for the heightened deep tendon and plantar reflexes on the left side of the body. Possibly, earlier transient ischemic attacks may have resulted in lacunar infarctions to the right cerebral hemisphere that were not visible on the CT scan. A repeated CT scan, approximately six weeks thereafter, showed no significant changes.

Finally, Mr. R.'s response latency continued to spontaneously diminish with time. Currently, he exhibits only slight delays (1–2 seconds) when interacting with another person during conversation.

REFERENCES

Ardila, A., & Lopez, M.V. (1984). Transcortical motor aphasia: One or two aphasias? *Brain and Language, 22*(2), 350–353.

Damasio, H. (1981). Cerebral localization of the aphasias. In M. T. Sarno (Ed.), *Acquired aphasia.* New York: Academic Press.

Goodglass, H., & Kaplan, E. (1983). *The assessment of aphasia and related disorders.* Philadelphia: Lea and Febiger.

Luria, A.R. (1966). *Higher cortical functions in man.* New York: Basic Books.

Myers, P.S. (1984). Right hemisphere impairment. In A. Holland (Ed.), *Language disorders in adults.* San Diego: College-Hill Press.

Myers, P.S. (1986). Right hemisphere communication impairment. In R. Chapey (Ed.), *Language intervention strategies in adult aphasia* (2nd ed.). Baltimore: Williams & Wilkins.

Solomon, S. (1985). Application of neurology to psychiatry. In H.I. Kaplan & B.J. Sadock (Eds.), *Comprehensive textbook of psychiatry* (4th ed.). Baltimore: Williams & Wilkins.

INTERMITTENT PURE-WORD DEAFNESS?

*W*hile the accurate diagnosis of a speech–language disorder is often consuming and demanding, it is a necessary and integral part of the overall management of the patient by all health-care professionals involved. The evaluation of communication disorders secondary to a neurological etiology is predicated on conceptual knowledge of speech and language mechanisms and a practical approach to assessing the integrity of those mechanisms. The differential diagnosis of a neurogenic communication disorder is not carried out in isolation. Instead, the information gleaned by the speech–language pathologist must be coupled with medical and neuropsychological data in order to establish the most accurate diagnosis.

BRIEF CASE HISTORY

Our patient, Mr. K., was a 68-year-old, right-handed man who was in a normal state of health until the day of admission. A high school graduate, Mr. K. was a retired farm equipment operator and lived alone without difficulty. He was born and lived his entire life in the Midwest.

On the day following his admission, a Neurology resident sent Speech Pathology service a consult that simply read:

Reason for request: "Defication of speech"

In addition to providing us with our daily dose of humor, the consult introduced us to one of the most interesting cases we have seen. Review of Mr. K.'s medical record indicated a history of hypertension and various minor medical problems of no apparent consequence to the current admission. The record revealed that he was brought to the hospital by his daughter, who described her father as disoriented with rambling, nonsensical speech. CT scans obtained on the day of admission were normal, as were motor signs. Despite the lack of CT evidence, Neurology service concluded, on the basis of language disorder, that Mr. K. suffered a probable left temporoparietal infarct.

Our initial bedside evaluation found Mr. K. sitting in a wheelchair gazing out his hospital window. When we greeted him he just sat looking out the window without observable recognition that someone wanted to interact with him. After getting his attention, however, we found him to be highly fluent with intact speech, but unable to follow even one-part auditory commands. In many ways he behaved as if he were severely hard of hearing or deaf, or that his native English sounded like a foreign language. His speech output was phonologically and syntactically accurate. It was object- but not task-specific. Mr. K. would freely discuss objects when they were present, but without the object in place his speech became non–task-specific. No literal or verbal paraphasic errors were noted. He would soliloquize at length about the weather, the hospital, his family and work with no apparent need for input from the listener. Effective interactive communication could be achieved only when all input directed toward him was written. Using written directions, we were able to complete a screening of reading, writing, and naming skills. This limited sample suggested that the patient was having no significant difficulties on these tasks. It became apparent during this bedside evaluation that a comprehensive assessment would be required in order to establish an accurate diagnosis and implement appropriate treatment.

SUBSEQUENT EVALUATION

As we began exploring Mr. K.'s communication problems in more depth, some very informative, but at times confusing, evidence emerged. For example, the medical record of the night before indicated that his symptoms had cleared and he was back to a normal baseline, but that was not what we found on the second day. Instead, the profound auditory processing deficit seen during the bedside exam persisted and the patient again could not follow even the simplest of auditory commands. Interestingly, there was a nurse's note made on the morning of our evaluation that stated the patient was experiencing an increased heart rate at approximately 155 beats per minute. The patient was treated with digoxin, and a cardiology consult was sent.

Despite the fluctuating physical condition, over the next two days we administered the following tests:

- The Western Aphasia Battery (Kertesz, 1982)
- Boston Naming Test (Kaplan, Goodglass, & Weintraub, 1983)
- Revised Token Test (McNeil & Prescott, 1978)
- Reading Comprehension Battery for Aphasia (LaPointe & Horner, 1979)
- Porch Index of Communicative Ability—Graphic Subtests (Porch, 1967)
- A full audiometric evaluation.

When directions were presented to the auditory modality alone the patient was unable to be tested reliably; he consistently stated he didn't know what we wanted of him. Repetition of an instruction was unsuccessful in eliciting task-related performance. Instead, we had to administer all tests with written instructions, except, of course, the evaluation of auditory comprehension, which was profoundly impaired. With written instructions, the patient demonstrated intact speech–language oral expression, as well as intact reading, writing, orientation, and memory of recent and distant events. His only verbal output problem appeared to be mild anomia in spontaneous speech and a tendency to discuss topics without specific information related to the target topic.

Mr. K. then began a series of psychiatric, radiological, and audiological evaluations. Psychiatry service stated that the patient was not testable due to his noncompliant behaviors in the test environment. They did conclude that Mr. K. appeared senile and that nursing home placement should be explored, as independent living was no longer possible. Radiology service repeated CT scans, which again showed no lesion. The audiological evaluation indicated no peripheral and/or brainstem involvement. Speech detection thresholds were at 10 and 12 dB HL with brainstem auditory evoked responses (BAER) within normal limits.

This patient's severe auditory processing difficulties persisted, so we began to examine his auditory system in greater detail. Using audiotapes of 40 familiar nonlinguistic sounds (Finitzo-Hieber, Matkin, Cherow-Skala, & Gerling, 1977), ranging from doors slamming to water dripping, we found that the patient could effectively process nonverbal environmental sounds. We then compared his ability to process environmental sounds to his ability to process language using random presentation; Mr. K. responded with 90 percent accuracy for nonlinguistic but only 5 percent accuracy for linguistic information. Furthermore, using procedures established by Ross (1981) this patient showed no difficulty with prosodic–affective comprehension or comprehension of emotional gesturing.

A new review of Mr. K.'s medical record again showed that after his evening meal he experienced a remission of his symptoms lasting throughout the night. He could understand speech without difficulty, and his spontaneous speech was described as informative. EKG results, on that day, indicated the patient to be experiencing atrial fibrillation with rapid ventricular response. Since his behaviors were fluctuating so rapidly with what seemed to be a paralleling cardiac status, the main focus in this acute stage was to stabilize the patient medically. In addition to the digoxin, Mr. K. was given Quinidine to control his fibrillations. At this point we were ready to make a diagnosis and suggest follow-up management.

DISCUSSION

While this patient's speech and language problems appeared to be directly attributable to his cardiac difficulties (specifically, transient atrial fibrillation lasting two to five hours), it was important for us to describe the speech and language problems as a baseline against which his subsequent behaviors could be compared. It was also important for us to make recommendations for communicating with the patient when he was experiencing difficulties.

From the onset it was clear that bypassing this patient's auditory modality resulted in near normal language functioning, with the exception of a mild anomic component. We began exploring agnosia as a possible underlying reason for his observed behaviors. When written instructions preceeded all required tasks, Mr. K.'s speech and language skills were easily within normal limits, and his output became relevant to the topic. The anomic component did not appreciatively interfere with effective communicative functioning. The striking language comprehension deficit appeared to have no peripheral or central nervous system component, nor was it caused by a sensory hearing loss. Furthermore the patient could respond correctly to environmental sounds. Our assessing the integrity of Mr. K.'s auditory system, and then bypassing it in an effort to ascertain the nature of his disorder, reflected concepts presented by Brookshire (1986). He suggested that prior to establishing a diagnosis of agnosia or related disorders, one must first exclude four possibilities. (Given the fluctuating nature of the disorder, we added a fifth possibility to the list.)

1. Sensory deficits in the affected modality
2. Comprehension deficit
3. Expressive disturbance
4. Unfamiliarity with the test stimulus
5. Psychiatric disturbance

SENSORY DEFICITS

Based on audiometric test results, Mr. K. demonstrated an intact auditory peripheral system without brainstem involvement. In addition, this patient was able to respond accurately and efficiently to nonlinguistic auditory information. Thus, we ruled out hearing loss as a possible cause of the observed behaviors.

COMPREHENSION DEFICIT

Because Mr. K. responded accurately to all our language tasks when the instructions were presented by means of other stimulus modalities, we eliminated a general intellectual deficit as an etiology to explain his input problems. Mr. K. had no difficulty understanding the written instructions to any and all tasks required of him.

EXPRESSIVE DISTURBANCE

Mr. K.'s speech and language output skills were consistently within normal limits for phonology and syntax. When this patient was made to understand task requirements by bypassing auditory inputs, his semantic and pragmatic levels of language fell within normal limits. In all, Mr. K. did not reveal the speech–language problems typical of Wernicke's aphasia, transcortical sensory aphasia, or other aphasia syndromes associated with severe auditory comprehension deficits.

UNFAMILIARITY WITH TEST STIMULUS

Because Mr. K. had no difficulty with any stimuli when presented through modalities other than the auditory, we did not think that unfamiliarity with the material could account for the behavior.

PSYCHIATRIC DISTURBANCE

From the initial session we kept questioning this patient's psychological make-up, and we asked the obvious question, "Is this patient putting us on?" The Psychiatric consult did little to help us answer this question. More important was the fact that Mr. K. had no previous history of psychological or psychogenic problems and appeared genuinely concerned regarding his present condition. But at the same time he seemed unaware of the magnitude of the problem or the fluctuations in his behavior. He often stated that he wanted to leave the hospital, as he had work to accomplish and the hospital stay was interfering with his plans. Even so, it was impossible to eliminate the existence of a psychogenic disorder completely as a potential contributing factor.

After arriving at a diagnosis of agnosia it became imperative to further describe the type of agnosia Mr. K. was experiencing, as well as the underlying neuroanatomical correlates. By doing so we believed we could further understand this patient's behavior and assist in the overall medical team management of Mr. K.

An account of various auditory deficits provided us a framework by which to approach this complicated diagnostic task (Albert, Goodglass, Helm, Rubens, & Alexander, 1981). The first type of agnosia we considered was generalized auditory agnosia. By definition a patient with generalized auditory agnosia exhibits an inability to comprehend verbal or nonverbal information with intact auditory acuity. As Mr. K. demonstrated an excellent ability to process nonlinguistic information accurately, we discarded this diagnosis. Auditory sound agnosia, an inability to recognize nonspeech sounds, and cortical deafness, an unawareness of auditory stimuli, were also discarded, because Mr. K. continued to demonstrate the ability to identify environmental auditory stimuli. The remaining diagnosis was pure-word deafness, also called auditory verbal agnosia. Consistent with this diagnostic description, Mr. K. demonstrated an ability to process nonverbal nonlinguistic information, as well as emotional intent and prosody. His reading and writing skills were commensurate with his educational level. He was, however, unable to comprehend even simple verbal commands.

Our recommendations included a daily schedule of treatment and a suggestion that all input be presented to this patient through a multimodality input format with emphasis on visual stimulation. Specifically, we suggested that members of the health care team write out their wishes to Mr. K. and couple them with verbal and gestural input as well.

While all behavioral evidence pointed toward a diagnosis of pure-word deafness, the rarity of this condition in the clinical environment, and the somewhat transient presentation Mr. K. demonstrated, made us wonder about the underlying neurological mechanism that could account for the patient's condition. Pure-word deafness usually arises from bilateral lesions that disconnect Wernicke's area from the primary auditory cortex in both hemispheres. It is also possible for pure-word deafness to arise from unilateral lesions in the left temporal lobe (Kanter, Day, Heilman, & Gonzalez Rothi, 1986). This lesion spares the posterior portion of the superior temporal gyrus, but destroys both the left auditory radiation from Heschl's gyrus and the callosal fibers originating in the right temporal lobe, thereby isolating Wernicke's area from the auditory input. Our patient, however, showed no evidence of brain lesion, either unilateral or bilateral. Kanter and colleagues, however, described three cases in which transient pure-word deafness occurred following extracranial–intracranial bypass, resulting in delayed transient neurological dysfunction. Kanter and colleagues hypothesized that local vascular disturbances secondary to operative manipulation of the recipient vessel, or leakage of small amounts of blood around the anastomosis, could cause the pure-word deafness encountered in their three patients.

These cases may shed some light on our own patient. We theorized that if Mr. K. had a vascular stenosis of the blood vessels supplying the cortical middle and posterior temporal end artery branches of the middle cerebral artery, he could experience pure-word deafness symptoms secondary to a localized decrease in blood flow during his cardiac arhythmias. PET scanning, had it been accomplished, may have provided additional information regarding the underlying etiology of Mr. K.'s behaviors. While this is conjecture, it does attempt to explain the puzzling and atypical presentation of Mr. K.

References

Albert, M., Goodglass, H., Helm, N.A., Rubens, A., & Alexander, M. (1981). *Clinical aspects of dysphasia.* New York: Springer-Verlag.

Brookshire, R.H. (1986). *An introduction to aphasia.* Minneapolis: BRK Publishers.

Finitzo-Hieber, T., Matkin, N.D., Cherow-Skala, E., & Gerling, I.J. (1977). *Sound effects recognition test (SERT).* St. Louis, MO: Auditec.

Kanter, S.L., Day, A.L., Heilman, K.M., & Gonzalez Rothi, L.J. (1986). Pure word deafness: A possible explanation of transient deteriorations after extracranial-intracranial bypass grafting. *Neurosurgery, 18,* 186–189.

Kaplan, E., Goodglass, H., & Weintraub, S. (1983). *Boston naming test.* Philadelphia: Lea and Febiger.

Kertesz, A. (1982). *The western aphasia battery.* New York: Grune & Stratton.

LaPointe, L.L., & Horner, J. (1979). *Reading comprehension battery for aphasia.* Tigard, Oregon: C.C. Publications.

McNeil, M.R., & Prescott, T.E. (1978). *Revised token test.* Baltimore: University Park Press.

Porch, B.E. (1967). *Porch index of communicative ability.* Palo Alto, CA: Consulting Psychologists Press.

Ross, E.D. (1981). The aprosodias: Functional–anatomic organization of the affective components of language and the right hemisphere. *Archives of Neurology, 38,* 561–569.

CHAPTER 8
JAMES L. ATEN

"RULE OUT PSYCHOSIS, DEMENTIA, ORGANIC BRAIN SYNDROME"

*T*he events described in this chapter should remind us of our responsibility to educate our colleagues in other hospital services as to the nature of communication disorders and how these disorders may affect patients under their care. In managing this case, I learned several lessons: (1) that Psychiatry Service, in particular, must be taught that atypical or even bizarre communicative behavior is not necessarily a sign of psychiatric disease; (2) that it is essential to obtain as much of the medical and social history as possible for each patient; (3) that test scores may not predict the patient's capacity for independent living.

THE REQUEST FOR CONSULTATION

Our V. A. Medical Center Speech Pathology Clinic received a consult from the Inpatient Psychiatry Service requesting evaluation of a 67-year-old male patient (Mr. H.). He had been seen in the emergency room two days previously and subsequently referred to Psychiatry, which then obtained the patient's consent for a 72-hour "Voluntary Admission for Psychiatric Evaluation." Because the hospital must discharge a patient who does not consent to further hospitalization, Psychiatry was anxious for our opinion. The consult from Psychiatry described Mr. H. as "agitated and confused with aggressive and paranoid tendencies . . . speaking and acting bizarrely." Their differential diagnostic considerations included organic brain syndrome, dementia, monopolar affective disorder (manic phase), and character disorder. Psychiatry was encouraged to consult the Speech Pathology Clinic by a staff clinical psychologist with a background in linguistics and communicative disorders. The psychologist questioned the psychiatric etiology of the symptoms and believed the patient not to be severely demented.

INITIAL SPEECH AND LANGUAGE SCREENING

Understanding the urgency, we proceeded immediately to the locked psychiatry ward, taking along the necessary screening test materials. A brief review of the medical chart revealed essentially no background information regarding Mr. H.'s social, vocational, or medical history, except for a vague reference to his having been admitted to a local hospital about one year previously. The chart indicated that the patient had arrived at the emergency room excitedly gesturing to his eyes and talking in words that no one could understand. He reportedly became increasingly agitated and frustrated as emergency room personnel failed to understand him. With that he was placed in a locked room, and when he attempted to leave was labeled "aggressive with combative tendencies."

Our initial contact with Mr. H. was on the ward at a table where he was seated looking at a newspaper. He smiled, stood up and greeted us with a self-conscious graciousness and jargon phrases. Interspersed with the paraphasic output were intelligible, socially appropriate utterances, such as "Hello, how are you?" Language screening materials were introduced along with nonverbal instructions and modeled response demonstrations, and the patient was able to show us that he

- Cooperated well once he was *shown*, as opposed to being told, what it was we wanted him to do
- Could match some short, familiar printed words with the appropriate pictured objects or actions with better than chance accuracy
- Could write recognizable parts of his name and copy most of his address using his dominant right hand
- Could select correct patterns from sampled Ravens Coloured Progressive Matrices Test (Ravens, 1962) items, suggesting a degree of functional capacity in the nonverbal sphere
- Could not follow commands delivered orally, nor comprehend names of objects, actions, colors, or forms.
- Could not comprehend familiar spoken words that he read correctly.

These preliminary test results and observations led to the following recommendations:

1. Immediately attend to his right eye infection in response to the complaint that originally brought him to the medical center
2. Conduct a hearing test as soon as possible
3. Obtain additional case history information
4. Request that Mr. H. be released from the locked ward and monitored for compliance with scheduled tests
5. Administer more extensive and comprehensive language and nonverbal tests

CASE HISTORY INFORMATION

After our first contact with Mr. H., a phone call to the friend whose name had appeared in the medical chart provided the following information. Mr. H., who had no immediate family, had retired several years prior from a successful career as a postal worker. In the years since his retirement he lived alone pursuing several hobbies, including fishing, until he experienced a left hemisphere stroke. He had recovered physically from that stroke, and within two weeks of its occurrence left a private hospital against medical advice. For one year he lived alone, but got along quite well with the help of a friend and a public health nurse who helped him with antiseizure medications. The friend helped him pay his bills from his retirement income and have adequate cash available to purchase food and pay the rent. The friend, who owned a charter boat, also took him fishing quite often. Our patient's life had been relatively pleasant and uneventful until he sought treatment for his eye infection at the emergency room.

TEST RESULTS

Additional speech and language testing was conducted in the Speech Pathology Clinic over the next few days. No single test could be administered completely (see Behavior During Testing section below). The scores on subtests that were obtained confirmed our initial impressions from the screening on the ward, which was that Mr. H. was neither psychotic nor demonstrating evidence of a global cognitive deficit.

AUDIOLOGICAL ASSESSMENT

Audiometric testing determined that hearing for speech (speech detection thresholds) was at the 30 dB level bilaterally, and variable pure-tone threshold responses indicated "a mild hearing loss through the speech range — at most."

TESTS FOR APHASIA

The language assessment included administrations of portions of the following formal and informal tests:

- Boston Diagnostic Aphasia Exam (BDAE) (Goodglass & Kaplan, 1983)
- Porch Index of Communicative Ability (PICA) (Porch, 1967)
- Ravens Coloured Progressive Matrices (RCPM) (Ravens, 1962)
- Experimental editions of phonemic and semantic single and paired words contrasting auditory and reading discrimination-recognition-association
- Assessment of Children's Language Comprehension (ACLC) (Foster, Giddan, & Stark, 1973)

BEHAVIOR DURING TESTING

Mr. H. initially could tolerate testing for only brief periods because he frequently did not understand the task presented and demonstrated a limited attention span. His responses to modality specific tasks confirmed the impression from the earlier screening, that he responded best with visual stimuli such as printed words. He could copy printed material and correct errors in spontaneously written productions of his address when cued by the examiner. Responses to printed commands and statements were far superior to his responses to spoken stimuli. In fact, his most consistent area of deficit was a profound loss of ability to respond to spoken words, commands, or conversational information, combined with little or no awareness of his listening problems. This latter problem is comparable to anosognosia, seen frequently in patients with posterior right hemisphere lesions, who fail to appreciate the presence or severity of their left-sided motor deficits. Mr. H. responded to auditory stimulation of any type with self-conscious smiling or chuckling and would often begin talking simultaneously with the examiner. Obviously, this created problems in administering and completing formal tests. Gesturing or written stimulation, on the other hand, never evoked such a response.

SPEECH AND LANGUAGE TEST RESULTS

The PICA auditory subtests revealed very poor auditory comprehension for descriptive function phrases (Test VI = 6.5/15) and only fair comprehension of the names of objects (Test X = 11.2/15). The latter result was comparable to the score on the BDAE auditory discrimination subtest (22/72) and Test A of the ACLC (5/11). Mr. H. read and associated single words with pictures with approximately 50 percent accuracy, but consistently performed better when geographical names were used as stimuli with a map for responding (see Table 8-1). He was unable to read aloud or perform oral repetition tasks. Spontaneous speech consisted of jargon (i.e., verbal paraphasias) and neologisms, and an absence of contentive words when propositional language was attempted. Informal, casual, or reactive speech was marked with "islands" of fluent, intelligible over-learned words and phrases. The pattern of severe auditory comprehension deficits with slightly better reading ability, jargon, and paraphasic but fluent speech production was compatible with a diagnosis of Wernicke's aphasia.

NONVERBAL ASSESSMENTS

The only formal measure administered to estimate nonverbal cognitive functioning was the Ravens Coloured Progressive Matrices test, on which he scored 18/36, or slightly above the twenty-fifth percentile compared to normal healthy adults. When this performance was considered in conjunction with his ability to produce graphic figures to convey information when gestures failed, his excellent visuospatial orientation, and his capacity for independent living, we believed that dementia was not an appropriate primary diagnosis.

CT SCAN

Figure 8-1 depicts the CT scan obtained several months after our initial contact at approximately 17 months after his cerebrovascular accident. The scan was read as essentially unchanged from the one taken by the private

TABLE 8-1.
Initial speech/language test results.

Measure	Result
Porch Index of Communicative Ability	
Test VI (Auditory by function)	6.5/15
Test X (Auditory by name)	11.2/15
Boston Diagnostic Aphasia Examination	
Auditory discrimination (word recognition)	22/72
Assessment of Children's Language	
Comprehension	
Test A	5/16
Ravens Coloured Progressive Matrices	
Tests A, Ab, B	18/36
Informal Reading Tasks	
Picture-Word matching	50%
Geographical names map	80%
Informal Writing Tasks	
Spontaneous printing name (right hand)	100%
Spontaneous production of address	60%

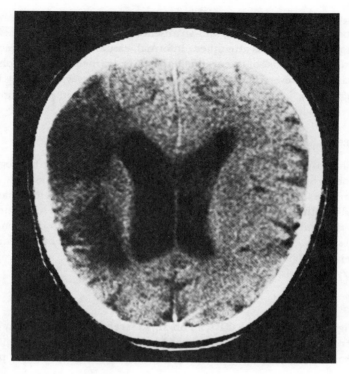

Figure 8-1. CT scan of patient H. at 17 months post-CVA. Reveals a large infarct in left temporal-parietal area.

hospital at about 10 days after the stroke. It showed "a large infarct in the (L) temporal-parietal area, including the superior posterior temporal lobe. There is considerable dilation of the left temporal horn possibly involving the isthmus. Some atrophy exists in the insula and there is moderate but within-normal limits atrophy in the (R) temporal area."

The documentation of the lesion supported the clinical diagnosis of Wernicke's aphasia. The site and extent of the lesion, as well as the degree of recovery, made this patient comparable to those patients reported by Naeser and colleagues (1987), who showed no recovery of sentence-level auditory comprehension. That group of patients similarly infarcted more than one-half of their superior posterior temporal gyri.

DISCHARGE

Psychiatry accepted the diagnosis of Wernicke's aphasia, obtained medical treatment for Mr. H.'s eye infection, and approved plans to discharge the patient with the recommendation that he come for speech and language treatment as an outpatient. Mr. H. seemed to understand our desire to have continued contact with him, while at the same time he wholeheartedly endorsed the opportunity to return home to his pre-admission lifestyle. Twice-weekly speech therapy appointments were established, and Mr. H. agreed to travel to the hospital by bus.

SPEECH AND LANGUAGE TREATMENT OVERVIEW

Therapy was initiated on a biweekly basis and continued for eight months. Attendance was sporadic because Mr. H. sometimes took unplanned and unannounced vacations, scheduled fishing trips that took precedence over treatment, or occasionally forgot to consult his list of appointments. The goals of treatment were partly in keeping with principles stated by Kennedy (1983):

> Patients (Wernicke's) who have little or no ability to recognize and comprehend auditory stimuli and who are not aware of their speech difficulties are not candidates for intensive and direct language treatment intervention. Intervention . . . must emphasize improvement of communication. (p. 18)

Treatment procedures included:
- Improving attention to printed requests for information
- Using cards in his wallet to answer questions and alert the listener to his problems
- Writing his name and address on forms
- Using a map to indicate birthplace and places he lived or worked
- Reducing the amount of jargon speech by substituting cued, short word and phrase answers to simultaneously spoken *and* written requests
- Accepting cues from his clinician to be quiet and attend to various inputs while delaying his responses

RESPONSE TO TREATMENT

After eight months of treatment Mr. H. had not improved in ability to process spoken words or conversation. Various measures of auditory processing remained at the twenty-fifth to twenty-seventh percentile level. Comprehension of sentences as measured by the Auditory Comprehension Test for Sentences (Shewan, 1979) revealed a score of 6/21, or 29 percent. Reading of single words remained higher than auditory recognition (fifty-fifth to sixtieth percentile correct), but functional reading as measured on the Reading Comprehension Battery for Aphasia was only 10 percent accurate. When the same lexical items were both written and spoken, Mr. H.'s performance improved to over 80 percent accuracy. Repeated observation of Mr. H.'s medical center attendance record for appointments validated our clinical impressions that transmitting information to him by both speaking and writing was preferred.

Mr. H.'s ability to speak, beyond socially appropriate greetings, did not become functional for communication. Jargon and verbal paraphasias persisted in his oral responses. Direct therapy attempts to facilitate naming, oral repetition, and imitation only served to shift Mr. H. from fluent output to hesitant, labored struggle with less recognizable, distorted productions. As a whole, he found such tasks frustrating and confusing, and responded with self-conscious laughter and a request to terminate the therapy session. Indirect stimulation using maps, magazine pictures of historical events, and geographic locales that were personally relevant, evoked fluent phrases that over time increased in length and substantive content, as noted in Table 8-2. These fluent, prosodically normal, highly intelligible "islands of fluency" could not be voluntarily produced. We tried writing down all spontaneous "real word" utterances and asked him to read them aloud, following the example of Helm and Barresi (1980), but this was not productive because his ability to read aloud was only minimally intact. Writing single spontaneous words to convey meaning did show some mild improvement during the treatment period and, along with gesture, became the main modalities of expression.

DISCUSSION

What overall lessons does this patient's early mismanagement have for us? Benson (1979) has commented that Wernicke-type aphasic patients are too often misdiagnosed and committed to psychiatric wards or mental

TABLE 8-2.
Mr. H.'s indirectly evoked utterances at two different stages in therapy.

Earlier in Treatment	Later in Treatment
It's O.K.	Yeah, that guy right up there
Right here	I remember that
All the way down	That's a Russian
Oh yeah	This one — I forgot his name
That's right	You had to hide [bomb exploding]
I don't see nothing	He's no good [picture of Hitler]
See up here	She died
Let's see	He goes over to his brother's

institutions. Tonkonogy (1986), in describing posterior-lesioned aphasias, states "patients . . . are often unaware that they have a language disorder and become very angry and agitated when someone fails to understand them" (p. 90). Even after treatment, when we or others used spoken language as the major means of communicating with him, Mr. H. showed what could be termed "bizarre behavior." This was minimized when writing and gestures were used. Certainly we have a continued obligation to remind ourselves, and to educate other professionals to recognize, that communication is not limited to verbal exchange. Furthermore, we have an obligation to inform physicians and other medical personnel of the behavioral characteristics of Wernicke's aphasia. In-service education could provide videotaped examples of Wernicke's patients who have great difficulty producing and understanding spoken language but otherwise are able to manage in their daily activities.

Health care providers must be instructed to explore writing as an alternative means of communication with patients who fail to respond to the spoken word. Furthermore, when a self-referred patient presents with a severe communication problem, Speech and Language Pathology and Neuropsychology should be considered immediately.

Conclusions

This case reminds us, first, that nothing can substitute for a complete case history. A single phone call to the friend named in the medical chart would have prevented an inappropriate initial placement. Mr. H. never forgot his "voluntary" confinement and the initial failure to treat the eye condition for which he sought help. His forceful gestures with fist clenched in the direction of the locked ward followed by pointing to his eye and shrugging his shoulders provided nonverbal expression of his feelings about the incident. Case history information should be combined with careful exploration of all possible etiologies and consultation with other services where indicated.

A final lesson from our case relates to treatment expectations. While the Speech Pathology Clinic's treatment did not result in significant improvements in speech and language, it did improve communication and relieve agitation and frustration. Treatment shifted from what Wertz (1983) terms a "curing" orientation to a "caring" one by becoming a valuable resource for our patient. Whenever he needs help with medical appointments or with medication directions, he has learned to come to the Speech Pathology Clinic before he goes elsewhere in the medical center. We decipher his needs and often write out messages he can take to other clinics and caregivers in the hospital. He now wears a badge informing others, "I have trouble understanding spoken messages — please write things down." Furthermore, we sometimes are called upon to act as interpreters when he unsuccessfully tries to negotiate the medical system on his own.

ACKNOWLEDGMENTS

Thanks are expressed to the Long Beach Veterans Administration Medical Center for support in preparation of this chapter. Gratitude is also owed to Dr. Susan Houston, neuropsychologist, who referred Mr. H. to Speech Pathology, and to clinicians Sydelle Rennick and Jamie Larson, who provided speech treatment for Mr. H. and maintained records of his responses.

REFERENCES

Benson, D.F. (1979). *Aphasia, alexia, and agraphia*. New York: Churchill Livingston.

Foster, R., Giddan, J., & Stark, J. (1973). *Assessment of children's language comprehension*. Palo Alto, CA: Consulting Psychologists Press.

Goodglass, H., & Kaplan, E. (1983). *The assessment of aphasia and related disorders* (2nd ed.). Philadelphia: Lea and Febiger.

Helm, N., & Barresi, B. (1980). Voluntary control of involuntary utterances: A treatment approach to severe aphasia. In R. Brookshire (Ed.), *Clinical aphasiology conference proceedings*. Minneapolis: BRK Publishers.

Kennedy, J.L. (1983). Treatment of Wernicke's aphasia. In W. Perkins (Ed.), *Language handicaps in adults*. New York: Thieme-Stratton Inc.

Naeser, M., Helm-Estabrooks, N., Haas, G., Auerbach, S., & Srinivasan, M. (1987). Relationship between lesion extent in Wernicke's area on computed tomographic scan and predicting recovery of comprehension in Wernicke's aphasia. *Archives of Neurology, 44*, 73-82.

Porch, B. (1967). *The Porch index of communicative ability*. Palo Alto, CA: Consulting Psychologists Press.

Ravens, J. (1962). *Ravens coloured progressive matrices*. London: H.K. Lewis

Shewan, C.N. (1979). *Auditory comprehension test for sentences (ACTS)*. Chicago: Biolinguistics Clinical Institute.

Tonkonogy, J.M. (1986). *Vascular aphasia*. Cambridge, MA: MIT Press.

Wertz, R.T. (1983). Language intervention context and setting for the aphasic adult: When? In J. Miller, D. Yoder, & R. Schiefelbusch (Eds.), *Contemporary issues in language intervention* (ASHA Reports 12). Rockville, MD: American Speech-Language-Hearing Association.

CHAPTER 9

NANCY DREW

<hr/>

WERNICKE'S APHASIA
WITHOUT SITE
OF LESION
CONFIRMATION?

*T*he mysteries of the mind are bewildering even to the most experienced detectives and clinicians. What appears to be obvious is sometimes not substantiated by the evidence.

On September 12, 1985, we received a consult from the Inpatient Neurology Service stating "68 yr. old male with aphasia and right-sided hemiparesis secondary to probable left hemisphere stroke last Sunday (9/8/85). Please evaluate."

MEDICAL HISTORY

The medical chart notes on this 68-year-old man, Mr. F., read as follows:

9/8/85–Patient admitted to St. Luke's Hospital at which time he "appeared to be drunk" and made no sense.

9/10/85–Patient transferred to San Francisco Veterans Administration Hospital Medical Center with the following symptoms: right-sided hemiparesis of the face, arm and leg, with right-side hyperreflexia, left irregular pupil and no visual field cuts. His speech was limited to short phrases such as "fine, thanks." He was noted to have severe auditory comprehension difficulty.

9/11/85-CT scan without contrast reveals a patchy, low density area in the anterior portion of the middle temporal gyrus (anterior and inferior to Wernicke's area). An additional small lesion is present lateral to the left occipital horn possibly interrupting the fibers of the optic radiations as well as fibers from auditory contralateral pathways.

9/13/85-CT scan with contrast shows a small, patchy, low density area in the anterior portion of the middle temporal gyrus. An additional small, low density area is present lateral to the left occipital horn with small superior extension deep to the posterior supramarginal gyrus. There is no area of enhancement seen on this scan.

9/20/85-MRI scan was done with T1 and T2 weighted axial images. Both the T1 and T2 weighted images revealed an area of hyperintensity lateral to the left occipital horn. In addition, there are multiple, bilateral, small, high signal intensity foci throughout the periventricular white matter and centrum semiovale. "None of these lesions is associated with any mass effect of hemorrhage. The appearance is most suggestive of subcortical arterioslerotic encephalopathy (SEA)." The small anterior middle temporal gyrus lesion present on the previous 2 CT scans is not visualized on the present MRI scan.

10/2/85-CT scan without contrast reveals only a very small, patchy low density area lateral to the left occipital horn (present on one slice only).

Within a week, the right-sided hemiparesis had almost completely resolved, but the Wernicke's aphasia remained the prominent symptom. The question was, Why did Mr. F. have such a fairly clear Wernicke's syndrome without supporting CT scan evidence of cortical damage to Wernicke's area or subcortical damage to the auditory pathways of the temporal isthmus? Normally one would expect to see a lesion in the posterior two-thirds of the superior temporal gyrus of the left hemisphere (Albert, Goodglass, Helm, Rubens, & Alexander, 1982), or in the subcortical temporal isthmus (Ti) (Naeser, Alexander, Helm-Estabrooks, Levine, Laughlin, & Geschwind, 1982). The Ti is a small subcortical area extending from the posterior and inferior portion of the sylvian fissure across to the temporal horn. The anterior half of the Ti carries auditory fibers from the medial geniculate nucleus of the thalamus out to Heschl's gyrus. Interruption of these auditory pathways at the level of the Ti produces a language profile similar to that of a traditional Wernicke's aphasia syndrome.

PERSONAL HISTORY

Mr. F.'s personal history was pieced together over time with his assistance using maps as cues as well as the patient's writing of single letters and/or numbers. He was born and raised in Missouri, where he completed high school. He served as a gunner on a B-17 during World War II and flew 35 missions over Germany. After the war he worked in California in a saw mill until 1971, at which time he became a caretaker at a YMCA camp until his retirement in 1981. He never married, and years before had lost track of his two sisters. His joy was going to the library every day, where he read newspapers from around the world and became an expert on Africa. He knew the details of the political and social evolutions of every country on that continent.

INITIAL SPEECH AND LANGUAGE TESTING

The following diagnostic instruments were used: Boston Diagnostic Aphasia Exam (BDAE) (Goodglass & Kaplan, 1983); Boston Naming Test (BNT) (Kaplan, Goodglass, & Weintraub, 1983); Ravens Coloured Progressive Matrices (Raven, 1962); Reading Comprehension Battery for Aphasia (LaPointe & Horner, 1979); and an audiological examination. Throughout testing, Mr. F. was pleasant and cooperative.

AUDITORY FUNCTIONING

Mr. F. had a high frequency hearing loss above 3000 cps in his right ear. By his own report he had had no usable hearing in his left ear for many years. This was confirmed by his audiological exam. His hearing was adequate for face-to-face communication.

His scores on the BDAE were as follows: word discrimination and body parts — twenty-fifth percentile; commands and complex ideational — zero percentile.

On the Boston Naming Test he was not helped by phonemic cuing. In fact, verbal information appeared to confuse him. In group therapy, during the first months he could not follow conversations among several people. His chances of understanding were increased by calling his name to get his attention and insisting that he watch the speaker's face.

VISUAL AND READING FUNCTIONING

Mr. F. could not match printed words with pictures of objects, geometric forms, colors, or actions, although he did read and correctly identify *seven* by holding up seven fingers. Repeat testing showed improvement in reading at the single-word level. He scored 40 percent (4/10). His RCBA score was 49 percent and was administered in 40 minutes. Eight months later he scored 87 percent in only 17 minutes. On the Ravens he scored in the ninety-second percentile for his age group, showing that he could adequately perform a nonlinguistic, visual reasoning task. He needed only one escorted trip to the Speech Clinic to remember its location, which involves traversing a complex maze from his ward through three different buildings.

Speech and Language Functioning

Mr. F.'s speech was characterized by slow production with delays and repetitions of initial sounds and words, clear articulation, self-corrections, literal paraphasias, and neologistic jargon. Though fluent, his output was sparse and there was no "press of speech." The repetitions of sounds and words seemed to be more a word retrieval delay than palalalia (see Figure 9-1).

In conversation his sentence structure was complex and complete with accurate grammar. Oral peripheral exam was within normal limits, with the exception of the BDAE nonverbal agility subtest, on which he scored 80 percent. His automatic speech on initial testing was limited to "one, two, three, four, five." His repetition of single words was 30 percent. Oral reading of single words was 10 percent. BDAE Visual Confrontation Naming was 0 percent. Administration of the Boston Naming Test yielded a score of 23 percent (14/60). By presenting the phonemic cue visually (e.g., writing the first two or three letters of the word as underlined on the test) he could write and then orally read an additional 10 items, yielding a test score of 40 percent.

10/16/85

WONBEN...YES...TWO'S NEGS...WEAR...TOMORROW TO MEN YOUR HOURS...AND UP HERE. HEAD ALOW UP HERE. GIRL AND BOY GREWGBAD..BAD...BAD...MOD.MADAME..MOTHER..UH..BA. ..BAD.BAD...BEAD..NO..NO.......NO.

3/86

THE LADY IS BLIND. I THINK YOU TOLD ME. [He had remembered that the first sentence in the sentence dictation portion of the BDAE given a month earlier was "She can't see them."] SHE IS...AH...AH ...AM..MAKING A VERY..BAD..JOB..FOR..FOR..FOR..FOR..UM..UM.. WASHING FOR..FOR DISHES. THE..THE..THE..THE..THE..THE..UM ..BOY..BOY..BOY..F..BOY..UM...BOYS..UM..HE FINDS ON A..STOOL. HE'S..HE'S..UM..ABOUT READY TO..TO FIND HIM. HE IS FINDING COOKIES..COOKIES WHICH HE IS STEALING..STEALING..COOKIES ..COOKIES. THE GIRL IS HELPING..HELPING HIM AND UM.

Figure 9-1. Mr. F.'s verbal description of the Cookie Theft Picture.

GRAPHIC FUNCTIONING

Using his preferred right hand, Mr. F. could print his name and a portion of his address legibly. His effort to write "San Francisco" carried sufficient information for an intelligent guess as to the intent. By September 16th he scored in the fiftieth percentile on primer level writing, and in the seventy-fifth percentile (4/10) on spelling to dictation. His overall writing skills had improved to a level suggesting that this modality might serve as a means of communication.

SUMMARY

Mr. F. revealed an evolving Wernicke-like aphasia characterized by severely impaired auditory comprehension and relatively fluent, clearly articulated speech with literal paraphasias and jargon. Though reading and writing abilities initially were as severely impaired as auditory comprehension and verbal expression, they rapidly improved to a functional level and served as his major means of communicating during the first three months of his rehabilitation.

REEVALUATION

Following discharge from the hospital Mr. F. received daily intensive outpatient language therapy. The results of BDAE retesting in March of 1986 showed significant improvements in all modalities of language. Auditory comprehension for single words was in the ninetieth percentile, and in the eightieth percentile for commands and complex ideational material. His reading comprehension of single words was 100 percent. His comprehension of sentences and paragraphs was in the ninetieth percentile. His oral expression was fluent and grammatically accurate, but with delays and repetitions of short words and syllables when searching for words. He could repeat complex sentences accurately. He scored in the ninety-fifth percentile for the BDAE naming tasks. He scored 83 percent on the Boston Naming Test. A repeat of the RCBA showed his comprehension to be 84 percent in 14 minutes. Occasionally, however, he made critical functional reading errors such as checking "no" to the following two questions on an application to a State Veterans Home: "Are you a California resident? Any treatment at the VA or other hospital in the last 5 years?" We corrected these errors and in October of 1986 he moved to a Veterans Home where he continued language therapy. Mr. F. commuted to the San Francisco VA Hospital once a week for individual work using the computer and he attended communication group therapy.

Discussion

The patient's initial clinical presentation was difficult to characterize, but within a week evolved into a Wernicke-like syndrome. Because early CT scanning found no pathology in Wernicke's area or the temporal isthmus, confusion arose over the diagnosis. The behavioral picture did not fit with the site of his lesions. The neurologists were reluctant to call this Wernicke's-type aphasia because, according to CT scan, that area was spared. The CT scan and MRI scan did, however, reveal areas of damage in the anterior middle temporal gyrus and lateral to the left occipital horn, possibly interrupting fibers of the auditory contralateral pathways. This lesion combination could produce an initial, but probably not long-lasting, auditory comprehension deficit. Aphasia from this particular lesion profile is not frequently reported. The more common subcortical aphasia syndromes stem from lesions in the temporal isthmus, thalamus, putamen, caudate, and insular structures (Benson, 1979; Damasio, Damasio, Rizzo, et al., 1982; Naeser et al., 1982). It is important to remember, however, that lesions are not always visualized on CT scans obtained during the acute stage. Instead, the *behavior* of a patient, when seen acutely, may be a better guide for diagnosis and treatment. Subsequent MRI findings disclosed deep white matter lesions that did not include Wernicke's area. This white matter pathology interrupted the pathways to Wernicke's area and probably explains the initial speech and language findings. This particular type of subcortical aphasia, with such focal language findings, is uncommon.

Conclusion

The technology of CT scan and MRI are yielding more information about the brain and its complexities. The importance of on-going, in-depth language evaluation, which documents and communicates the rapid changes in language skills to the patient, family, and staff, is critical to ensure that the "medical evidence as to site of lesion" does not dictate how patients are approached. For example, only recently have some forms of subcortical aphasia been defined and classified. In the future we will probably identify still other syndromes. Until then we observe patients' behavior with the scrutiny of a private investigator and record our descriptions.

ACKNOWLEDGMENT

The author wishes to thank Carol Palumbo, Boston VAMC, and Jonathan Mueller, SFVA, for their assistance in interpreting the CT and MRI scans.

REFERENCES

Albert, M.L., Goodglass, H., Helm, N., Rubens, A., & Alexander, M. (1982). *Clinical aspects of dysphasia.* New York: Springer-Verlag.

Benson, D.F. (1979). *Aphasia, alexia, and agraphia.* New York: Churchill Livingston.

Damasio, A., Damasio, H., Rizzo, M., Varney, N., & Gersh, F. (1982). Aphasia with nonhemorrhagic lesions in the basal ganglia and internal capsule. *Archives of Neurology, 39,* 15-20.

Goodglass, H., & Kaplan, E. (1983). *The assessment of aphasia and related disorders* (2nd ed.). Philadelphia: Lea and Febiger.

Kaplan, E., Goodglass, H., & Weintraub, S. (1983). *The Boston naming test.* Philadelphia: Lea and Febiger.

LaPointe, L., & Horner, J. (1979). *Reading comprehension battery for aphasia.* Tigard, OR: C.C. Publications.

Naeser, M., Alexander, M., Helm-Estabrooks, N., Levine, H., Laughlin, S., & Geschwind, N. (1982). Aphasia with predominantly subcortical lesion sites. *Archives of Neurology, 39,* 2-14.

Raven, J.C. (1962). *Ravens coloured progressive matrices.* London: H. Lewis and Company.

SECTION IV

DIFFICULTIES IN CLASSIFYING APHASIA IN THE PRESENCE OF VISUOSPATIAL DISTURBANCE

CHAPTER 10

LESLIE J. GONZALEZ-ROTHI
TODD E. FEINBERG

"PATIENT WITH LEFT POSTERIOR CIRCULATION CVA, NOW WITH ANOMIC APHASIA. CAN YOU HELP?"

*O*ur Speech Pathology Service received a consult from Neurology which stated, "Patient with left posterior circulation CVA, now with anomic aphasia. Can you help?" The consult indicates that the posterior circulation is involved in this case, but no indication is given about whether this has been determined by anatomic study or by behavioral analysis of those behaviors presumed to be represented by the anatomic structures subserved by these arteries.

The posterior cerebral (PCA) arteries (left or right) are formed by the bifurcation of the basilar artery, with each PCA dividing into two main branches. The posterior temporal branch and its subdivisions supply the inferior surface of the temporal lobe, as well as the occipitoparietal and lingual gyri. The internal occipital branch and its subdivisions supply the medial aspect of the occipital lobes. In addition, branches of the PCA supply the thalamus, choroid plexus of the third ventricle, the lateral geniculate body, and some of the mesencephalon.

Knowing the structures supplied by these vessels, certain behaviors might be predicted to occur with infarctions of these vessels. Infarction in the distribution of the left PCA would induce a right homonymous hemianopia, alexia without agraphia, color agnosia, anomia, and memory deficits. Therefore, our initial diagnostic strategy is to assess whether our patient's symptoms match those which we would predict. If so, we confirm this for the physician and make a statement regarding prognosis for spontaneous recovery, the evolutionary pattern that recovery might take, and finally, whether treatment is indicated, and, if so, the nature of that treatment. If the symptoms do not match the suspected localization, an analysis of the underlying mechanism of the deficits will need to be explored.

PATIENT HISTORY

The patient, a 61-year-old, right-handed man with 11 years of education, had a complicated medical history. This history included two significant events: first, the sudden onset of a right visual defect, headache, and memory problems; and second, 22 days later, of right-sided neglect, right hemiparesis, apraxia, and aphasia (described as being able to say "only monosyllabic words"). The neglect and hemiparesis were noted to resolve. The patient was seen by us 58 days after the onset of initial symptoms and 36 days after the onset of the second set of symptoms.

The scant records indicated that the symptoms at onset were those expected from a posterior cerebral artery infarct, including memory problems and a visual deficit. However, the additional problems — neglect, hemiparesis, apraxia, and aphasia (other than the predicted anomic component) — occurring at 36 days were not explained by the posterior cerebral artery infarct. Also, CT scans performed on the day of admission as well as 10 and 38 days after the extension of symptoms, revealed no evidence of significant extension beyond the posterior cerebral artery distribution, with the lesion limited to the occipitotemporal junction (Figure 10-1). Certainly there was no explanation for any aphasia other than an anomia.

LANGUAGE PERFORMANCE

Table 10-1 reviews the patient's performance on the Western Aphasia Battery (WAB) (Kertesz & Poole, 1974). He was oriented, initiated conversation, and responded promptly to biographical questions. Utterances were easily and precisely articulated and of normal quantity. He spoke in phrases or short sentences, and with good use of functors, but few substantive words. When describing a picture, semantic paraphasias were common, and

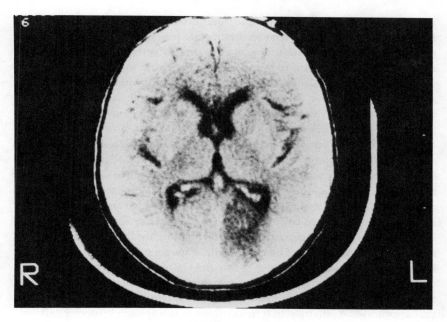

Figure 10-1. CT scan without contrast.

numerous pauses were noted at the points of major lexical items. Confrontation naming of pictures and held objects was profoundly impaired. While repetition was flawless, auditory comprehension was impaired. Although able to answer yes/no questions, his performance was significantly impaired on single word recognition tests and complex commands. In other words the configuration of this patient's performance on language testing was typical of that seen in cases of transcortical sensory aphasia.

To understand the mechanism of transcortical sensory aphasia we turned to Patterson and Shewell's (1987) language model in which three routes are

TABLE 10-1.
Western Aphasia Battery results.

Subtest	Patient Performance	TCS* Criteria
Fluency	6	5-10
Comprehension	5.56	0-6.9
Repetition	9.8	8-10
Naming	2.4	0-9

*TCS = transcortical sensory aphasia.

proposed for repeating words aloud; one nonlexical and two lexical (see Figure 10-2). It is thought that in the normal person each of these systems operates in parallel and simultaneously to process verbal information. The nonlexical route of repetition involves a direct acoustic-to-phonological conversion of verbal input without lexical or semantic mediation. Input is segmented, possibly at the level of the single phoneme, and converted to output. In contrast, for words that the person has previously experienced, the lexicon can be called upon to speed up this process. Two lexical systems are proposed. Both share an auditory input lexicon, which identifies input as familiar or not, possibly using phonological and syntactic information. Then, in the lexical semantic route, information about the word has access to meaning in the cognitive system. Subsequently, the person may verbally reproduce the stimulus word by means of the output lexicon. An alternative is the lexical-nonsemantic route. As with the lexical/semantic route, lexeme familiarity and phonological syntactic information are first achieved for the input in the input lexicon. Then the cognitive system is bypassed, with output lexicon providing whole-lexeme phonological information for output. Thus, only the lexical semantic route, allows us to apply meaning to what we hear, as well as to produce words meaningfully. It is this lexical semantic route that appears to be impaired in transcortical sensory aphasia involving deficits A or B in Patterson and Shewell's (1987) model. In this case the patient cannot

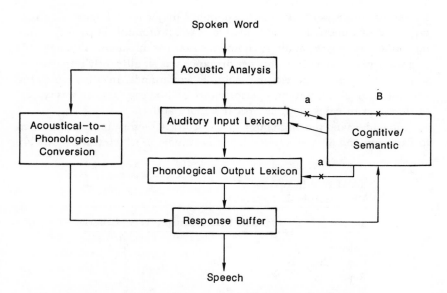

Figure 10-2. A portion of the Patterson and Shewell (1987) language model accounting for (A) repetition and (B) comprehension of auditorily received information.

apply meaning to what he or she hears or says, but repeats through the nonlexical or lexical-nonsemantic conversion. This explanation is compatible with the behavior of our patient, who had difficulty pointing to named objects, possibly suggesting an inability to link auditory input to meaning. In addition, he had word-finding difficulties, suggesting that he could not always retrieve from his lexicon on the basis of meaning. Yet he repeated, suggesting sparing of nonlexical and lexical-nonsemantic routes.

If the mechanism described above truly represents our patient's deficit, our treatments should address the inability to link meaning to words. Furthermore, if our patient has a disconnection between the cognitive system and input plus output lexicons (Figure 10-2A), treatment should emphasize pairing auditory input with another input modality, or verbal output with another output mode. In contrast, if our patient has a dysfunction of the cognitive system itself (Figure 10-2B), we should emphasize reconstruction of semantic relationships.

There are, however, some problems in applying these possible mechanisms to account for the syndrome of this case. For example, destruction of the semantic system requires large lesions not found in our neuroradiological data. In turn, the ability to link lexical phonology to meaning, as in the disconnection explanation we described above, requires disruption of temporal lobe outflow pathways. Again, this was not confirmed by CT. Only anomia was predicted by our patient's CT. However, it is not uncommon for the CT to be inconsistent with behavioral assessment in neurologically impaired patients. But as testing progressed, the diagnosis of transcortical sensory aphasia because less tenable.

GNOSIS

In reality, the patient's auditory comprehension was fairly good for biographical questions, review of factual information, and yes/no questions. In contrast, his auditory comprehension involving pointing commands using pictures or objects resulted in poorer performance. Although this behavior raised suspicion that the diagnosis of transcortical sensory aphasia was incorrect, it is not uncommon to see relatively better comprehension of yes/no questions or personal data questions in aphasic patients. As we watched the patient name objects, however, we became convinced that he did not recognize objects or pictures, although he consistently provided labels for each. Interestingly, he never complained of a difficulty recognizing pictures or objects. Was this object agnosia (failure to recognize the meaning of items perceived visually) as well as anomia? This diagnostic possibility was reduced by the fact that agnosia is most typically unimodal and results from bilateral lesions or extensive lesions of the left mesial occipital lobe (Bauer & Rubens, 1985). In our case his verbal or pantomime performance did not appear to improve with tactile or visual input, suggesting that his problem was multimodal. In addition, we saw only a unilateral left lesion of the inferior-medial occipitotemporal junction. However, we pursued this diagnostic possibility using tests of visual, tactile, and auditory gnosis, as well as copying visually presented material. The specifics of this evaluation are reviewed thoroughly elsewhere and the interested reader is referred to Feinberg, Rothi and Heilman (1986). For our differential diagnostic purposes here, it is most relevant to note that on further testing the patient matched objects visually, tactually, and cross-modally with 100 percent accuracy (see Table 10-2). But he was completely unable to provide any verbal or gestural information of any kind for those objects that he was able to match perfectly. In contrast, when given the name of these same objects verbally, the patient was able to describe or gesture their function, or point to the corresponding object, with at least 60 percent accuracy. This performance, though not normal, was significantly better than the patient's previous performances predicted. In other words, consistent with multimodal (visual/tactile) agnosia, the patient could give significantly more verbal or gestural information when items were named than when they were seen or felt.

Why does this distinction matter? We have reviewed treatments for transcortical sensory aphasia. What would we do differently with agnosia? In agnosia, unlike semantic dysfunction for a transcortical sensory aphasia, reconstruction of semantic relationships is not required. Instead the problem is the *linkage* of visually analyzed information to relatively *intact* semantic processes. In contrast to the case of the disconnection form of transcortical sensory aphasia, where we suggested using other input modalities to support audition, our strategy with this form of multimodal agnosia would be the use of audition to support visual and tactile inputs to meaning and slow removal of auditory support with time.

TABLE 10-2.
Agnosia test results.

Response (% correct)	Stimulus		
	Visual Object	Tactile Object	Name
Name	0	0	DNT*
Describe Function	0	0	70
Gesture	0	0	60
Visual Object	100	100	60
Tactile Object	100	100	DNT*

*DNT = did not test.

SUMMARY

In summary, we have described a case in which in addition to anomic aphasia characterized by poor word finding ability, we suspected multimodal (visual/tactile) associative agnosia characterized by the inability to gain meaning from visually or tactually presented objects. Using the WAB taxonomy, anomia and agnosia were misrepresented as transcortical sensory aphasia. It is interesting to note that Kertesz, Sheppard, and MacKenzie (1982), using the Western Aphasia Battery (Kertesz & Poole, 1974), also characterized patients with lesions similar to our patient's as transcortical sensory aphasia. One has to wonder if these patients also had multimodal (visual/tactile) associative agnosia mimicking transcortical sensory aphasia.

REFERENCES

Bauer, R.M., & Rubens, A.B. (1985). Agnosia. In K.M. Heilman & E. Valenstein (Eds.), *Clinical neuropsychology* (pp. 187-241). New York: Oxford University Press.

Feinberg, T.E., Rothi, L.J.G., & Heilman, K.M. (1986). Multimodal agnosia after unilateral left hemisphere lesion. *Neurology, 36,* 864-867.

Kertesz, A., & Poole, E. (1974). The aphasia quotient: The taxonomic approach to measurement of aphasic disability. *Canadian Journal of Neurological Science, 2,* 7-16.

Kertesz, A., Sheppard, A., & MacKenzie, R. (1982). Localization in transcortical sensory aphasia. *Archives of Neurology, 39,* 475-478.

Patterson, K., & Shewell, C. (1987). Speak and spell. In M. Coltheart, G. Sartori, & R. Job (Eds.), *The cognitive neuropsychology of language* (pp. 273-294). London: Lawrence Erlbaum Associates.

CHAPTER 11

KEVIN P. KEARNS
KATHERINE YEDOR

APHASIA COMPLICATED BY SEVERE VISUAL DEFICITS

CASE HISTORY

*M*r. S., a 67-year-old retired truck driver with a tenth grade education, was admitted to a local medical center on June 24, 1986 as a result of sudden onset of right hemiparesis and "transient" speech difficulties. Following a physical examination the admitting physician arrived at a provisional diagnosis of "expressive aphasia and right-sided hemiparesis secondary to a left hemisphere middle cerebral artery infarct." Mr. S. was subsequently transferred to the North Chicago VA Medical Center for further testing and treatment.

Mr. S.'s past medical history was positive for hypertension and chronic obstructive pulmonary disease. An intraocular lens was implanted following the removal of a cataract from his left eye. There were no previous reports of psychological or psychiatric disorders.

Prior to his hospitalization Mr. S. had been living alone, functioning independently, and appeared to be in good health. His stepdaughter reported, however, that his long-standing history of alcohol abuse had worsened over the previous six years, and there had been a noticeable decline in the patient's self care and personal hygiene over the previous several months.

CLINICAL OBSERVATIONS

Mr. S.'s medical records variously described him as disoriented, lethargic, and confused. Incidents of visual hallucinations also were documented, and he was reported to be agitated. He repeatedly removed his intraveneous line, so he was sedated and placed in soft restraints. He demonstrated various confabulatory behaviors; for example, when asked why he was in the hospital he stated that he had been involved in a "burn accident." Reports of confusion, disorientation, and agitation persisted for approximately 12 weeks.

TESTING

PHYSICAL AND NEUROLOGICAL EXAMINATION

Results of a neurological examination revealed that Mr. S. was disoriented to time and person, had reduced memory for recent events, aphasia, and confusion. A mild dysarthria and a right supranuclear facial palsy also were present, along with a right homonymous hemianopsia. A mild right-sided hemiparesis was reported. In addition, he had reported a right-sided hemisensory loss for superficial touch and, to a lesser extent, deep sensation and pain.

NEUROIMAGING

Magnetic Resonance Imaging (MRI) testing conducted three weeks after his cerebrovascular accident revealed "cerebral atrophy with a left posterior cerebral infarct." A CT scan conducted one week later confirmed the MRI results, and revealed a "recent infarction of the left posterior parieto-occipital region." An EEG obtained on the following day revealed abnormal slowing in the left hemisphere, especially in the temporal region.

INITIAL SPEECH/LANGUAGE CONSULTATION

At approximately three weeks post-onset, Mr. S. was seen at bedside for an initial speech–language evaluation. The examiner administered portions of the Boston Diagnostic Aphasia Examination (BDAE) (Goodglass & Kaplan, 1983) and an oral peripheral mechanism examination. Mr. S. was alert and cooperative during testing.

SEVERITY RATING

Mr. S. was assigned a rating of 2 on the BDAE Aphasia Severity Rating Scale. That is, "Conversation about familiar topics (was) possible with help from the listener. There (were) frequent failures to convey the idea, but the patient share(d) the burden of communication with the examiner."

CONVERSATIONAL AND EXPOSITORY SPEECH

During the Conversational and Expository Speech subtest of the BDAE, Mr. S. exhibited essentially normal fluency. That is, melodic line, phrase length, articulatory agility and grammatical form were unimpaired. His spontaneous speech was characterized by occasional semantic paraphasias, use of indefinite anaphoras, and circumlocutions.

AUDITORY COMPREHENSION

The initial attempt to administer the Word Discrimination subtest of the BDAE was discontinued. The examiner reported that Mr. S. "was unable to interpret pictured or printed stimuli." After discontinuing the subtest the examiner pointed to the picture of the chair and identified it, Mr. S. stated that it "looked like a ladder" to him.

On auditory comprehension subtests, where nearly all items did not require processing of visual stimuli, the patient's performance was moderately impaired. That is, he obtained scores of 14/20 on Body Part Identification, 10/15 for following auditory commands, and 5/12 on the BDAE Complex Ideational Materials subtest.

REPETITION

Performance on the BDAE repetition subtest was within normal limits. Mr. S. repeated the words and high probability phrases flawlessly. Similarly, he repeated six of eight low probability phrases without error. Minor paraphasic substitutions were produced on the final two low probability sentences (e.g., "soggy" for "foggy").

NAMING

Given Mr. S.'s strong negative reaction to tests involving visual stimuli, the Visual Confrontation Naming subtest of the BDAE was not administered. Performance on the Responsive Naming subtest resulted in a score of 26/30 (normal cutoff score is 27/30). On the Animal Naming subtest he named 6 animals in 60 seconds. (Suggested normal cutoff is 12; the standard deviation is 6.8.)

READING AND WRITING

Initial attempts to test reading were unsuccessful. The examiner reported that Mr. S. expressed "bewilderment and disbelief at his inability to interpret letters and words." While attempting the BDAE Word Reading subtest Mr. S. stated he could "see the letters in words" but could not read them, and he refused to attempt the reading tasks. Interestingly, he performed within normal limits on the BDAE Comprehension of Oral Spelling subtest (score of 7/8), a test that requires patients to identify words spelled orally by the examiner. Writing subtests were not attempted during the initial speech and language screening as soft restraints were in place during testing.

ORAL PERIPHERAL EXAMINATION

Positive findings on an oral peripheral mechanism examination included slightly reduced labial mobility, particularly on the left, and reduced breath support for speech. However, articulatory precision was judged to be within normal limits. Although Mr. S. was judged to be mildly dysarthric, there was a negligible interference with the intelligibility of spontaneous speech.

NEUROPSYCHOLOGICAL TESTING

During attempted administration of the Wechsler Memory Scale (Wechsler, 1945), Mr. S. was unable to interpret pictured and printed stimuli. He was disoriented to time and place (score was 1/11 for personal information and orientation subtests). When asked where he was, Mr. S. stated that he was in a "restaurant" rather than a hospital. This 67-year-old gentleman also stated that his age was "21 plus 2." An overall memory quotient could not be calculated for this "difficult-to-test" patient.

SUMMARY OF INITIAL IMPRESSIONS

Mr. S. exhibited a complex medical and behavioral history, and initial testing did not lead to a definitive diagnosis. For example, he had a long history of alcohol abuse in addition to his recent, sudden onset of neurological, language, and cognitive changes. In addition to his apparent language problems, he demonstrated disorientation, confusion, and management problems resulting from his state of agitation. Attempts at medical management, including sedation and physical restraint, further complicated the situation by affecting both his tolerance for testing and his test performances. Finally, the intial test results also were confounded by severe visual deficits of an unknown nature.

The results of language testing on the BDAE were consistent with a working diagnosis of "anomic" aphasia complicated by severe visual deficits and confusion of an unknown origin. In fact, his BDAE Rating Scale Profile of Speech Characteristics closely parallels the anomic profile presented and discussed by Goodglass and Kaplan (1983). Initial test results revealed a mildly impaired performance on responsive naming and a moderately severe anomic component on the BDAE animal naming test of word fluency. A moderately severe reduction in auditory comprehension was apparent for body-part identification and complex ideational material. Reading and writing were not tested. Severe visual deficits precluded processing of visuolinguistic information and a visual agnosia could not be ruled out on initial testing.

Following initial testing, Mr. S. received approximately three months of intermittent diagnostic therapy pending his ability to participate in more formal assessment. Sessions were limited in number during this period due to persistent confusion, disorientation, and agitation.

When Mr. S.'s confusional state began to resolve, formal testing was scheduled to obtain information relevant to the following diagnostic questions: (1) Did patient truly exhibit aphasia or should an alternate diagnosis, such as language of confusion, or language of generalized intellectual impairment, be entertained? (2) What was the nature of his visual deficit and how did it affect communication?

FOLLOW-UP SPEECH AND LANGUAGE TESTING

Approximately three months following the onset of his communicative deficits and the initial speech and language screening, Mr. S. finally was able to tolerate formal retesting. The BDAE was readministered, along with supplemental neuropsychological testing.

SEVERITY RATING

Mr. S.'s BDAE aphasia severity rating improved from 2 to 3, indicating that "the patient discuss(ed) *almost all everyday problems* with little or no assistance. Reduction of speech and/or comprehension, however, (made) conversation about certain material difficult or impossible."

CONVERSATIONAL AND EXPOSITORY SPEECH

Based on conversational and expository speech subtest of the BDAE, phrase length, fluency, grammar, melodic line, and articulatory agility were judged to be within normal limits. Paraphasias were not present in conversational speech. Information content was reduced in proportion to fluency and was characterized by frequent pauses prior to producing content words, indefinite anaphoras, and vague responses to questions. Numerous semantic paraphasias were frequently produced during the description of the cookie theft picture (for example, "water-keeper" for *sink*, and "basket" for *cookie jar*).

AUDITORY COMPREHENSION

Mr. S. performed within normal limits on BDAE auditory comprehension tasks that did not require reliance on visual skills. Specifically, he scored at or above the suggested cutoff scores for normal performance (Goodglass & Kaplan, 1983) on body-part identification (18/20), auditory commands (15/15), and the complex ideational material (8/12). By contrast, performance on the word discrimination subtest, a task that requires selection of visually presented materials, was moderately impaired (46/72). Many of his errors on this test (33%) were a result of response delays.

REPETITION

Repetition tasks were performed fluently and without error. Mr. S. flawlessly repeated all BDAE words, and high and low probability sentences.

NAMING

Mr. S. demonstrated only mild difficulties on the responsive naming subtest of the BDAE (26/30; normal cutoff is 27). His errors were due to one response delay and one verbal paraphasia (i.e., Q: "What do we cut paper with?" R: "knife"). More severe naming difficulties were demonstrated on the visual confrontation naming subtest (26/114). Mr. S. typically did not make any attempt to name pictured stimuli, often stating, "I'm gonna make a mistake and I don't want to." A few verbal paraphasias were produced during attempts to name numbers, and Mr. S. also perseverated on *watch* during this task. Phonemic cueing aided word retrieval during this subtest. On the Animal Naming (word fluency) subtest Mr. S. named 6 animals in 60 seconds, the same as before. During this subtest he commented, "I can think of 'em but I can't name 'em."

READING

Mr. S. was unable to orally read words or sentences. When attempting to read "triangle," he decoded "h-e-r" before giving up. Mr. S. was extremely sensitive about his reading difficulty, stating, "I can see it but I can't say it" and, "I'm just making a joke of myself." Matching letters and words was accomplished at chance levels of success. That is, he achieved a score of 4/10 on the Symbol and Word Discrimination subtest. On the Word Recognition subtest, a task that requires patients to point to words read aloud by the clinician, Mr. S. scored 6/8. He accurately recognized words spelled orally by the clinician (score was 8/8). However, he was unable to match words to pictures and stated that he was "guessing" (score was 0/10). The Reading Sentences and Paragraphs subtest was accomplished at chance levels of success (score was 2/10). The extent of his reading disability was further demonstrated later in the testing session by his *inability to read words that he had previously written*.

WRITING

Overall, Mr. S. received a scaled score of 4 for mechanics of writing, indicating that his cursive writing was legible but impaired. He received a raw score of 46 on Recall of Written Symbols, and he scored 14/15 on primer-level dictation. On the Spelling to Dictation subtest, he received a score of 8/10. On the written confrontation naming subtest, he received a score of 6/10. He produced minimal output with no legible information during a narrative writing task, but a score of 8/12 on writing sentences to dictation. Some visually based paragraphias were noted in this task (e.g., "streeting" for "stealing").

Supplemental testing showed that Mr. S. accurately copied a sequence of letters inserted within a task requiring him to replicate various geometric shapes. Interestingly, when asked to copy words of the same length, he initially produced illegible strings of unrelated letters and unrecognizable letter approximations. He subsequently refused to copy the remaining words, stating, "All the letters are the same" and, "They don't make any words at all."

TACTILE NAMING

Informal assessment of tactile naming was attempted to determine if Mr. S.'s anomic difficulties were also present in this modality. The clinician initially presented 10 common objects and asked the patient to name them. Based on visual input alone, he named 5 of the 10 objects. The patient was subsequently asked to close his eyes and name the same objects when they were placed in his right hand. He successfully named all ten objects through the tactile modality alone.

SUMMARY OF FOLLOW-UP SPEECH AND LANGUAGE TESTING

Three months after the initial bedside evaluation, Mr. S.'s confusional state resolved and more in-depth testing could be accomplished. Results of follow-up testing revealed adequate *auditory comprehension* for words, sentences, and paragraphs on tasks that required little or no visual processing. *Spontaneous speech* was well-articulated, grammatical, and fluent. Verbal agility, recitation of automatic sequences, and *repetition* of words and sentences were intact. However, responsive *naming* was mildly impaired and verbal fluency was one standard deviation below the normal cut-off score. Tactile naming was superior to visual naming of common objects. Performance on *oral reading* and *reading comprehension* tasks did not exceed chance levels of responding. *Writing* was functional, with errors produced for difficult words and sentences, and writing skills were far superior to reading. *In fact, when the examiner presented words previously written by the patient, he indicated that he was unable to read them.* While in the process of writing words legibly, Mr. S. stated that he was producing "scribbles."

NEUROPSYCHOLOGICAL TESTING

MEMORY AND ORIENTATION

On the Personal and Current Information and Orientation subtests of the Wechsler Memory Scale, Mr. S. scored 1/11. But, when the clinician verbally stated three alternate choices, Mr. S. immediately selected the correct answers to these same questions. On the Logical Memory subtest, he was only able to provide the main idea without any details of short paragraphs read to him (score of 1/23). He was able to repeat five digits in forward order and three digits in reverse order. Reproduction of geometric figures from memory was reduced (score was 6/23). Forms were generally complete, although lacking in some details and distorted in shape and size. No overall memory quotient was calculated for Mr. S., as the severity of his language deficits interfered with his performance on many subtests and reduced the validity of this measure.

VISUAL DISCRIMINATION

On subtests of the Frostig Developmental Test of Visual Perception (Frostig, 1966), Mr. S. was able to accurately complete tasks requiring visual discrimination of similar shapes and objects (raw score was 7/8 on subtest IV).

PARIETAL LOBE BATTERY OF THE BDAE

On the Drawing to Command subtest, Mr. S. received a raw score of 2/13. When given drawings to copy, his score improved to 9. On the stick construction from memory subtest, Mr. S. scored 5/14. When given a model to copy, his score improved by only 1 to 6. He received a score of 8/12 on the clock setting subtest, with errors due to failure to differentiate length of hands. On the calculation subtest, he received a score of 8 out of 32, although he was able to add up to four 2-digit numbers accurately.

DISCUSSION

The results of a speech and language screening examination administered three weeks after the onset of his deficits were consistent with a diagnosis of anomic aphasia complicated by severe visual deficits. These initial impressions could not be verified, refined, or altered for several months, as further testing could not be accomplished due to persistent confusion and disorientation. In addition, additional information regarding the nature of his visual impairment and its impact on language testing had to await additional testing.

While transient confusion and disorientation may be present following posterior cerebral artery (PCA) infarction (Devinsky, Bear, & Volpe, 1988), it is highly unusual for these symptoms to persist for several months, as they did with this patient. The persistence of Mr. S.'s confusional state led us to question whether he was truly aphasic. Consequently, alternative diagnoses, such as or "language of confusion" and "language of generalized intellectual impairment" (Wertz, 1985), were considered during the period of diagnostic therapy that occurred prior to formal testing. These alternatives were weighed in light of available case history information, neuroradiodiagnostic test results, and behavioral observations made during diagnostic therapy sessions.

Despite his disorientation and reported confusion, Mr. S. did not exhibit confused *language*. That is, he did not produce the irrelevant and tangential verbal output that is characteristic of this diagnosis. Furthermore, confabulation, another hallmark of patients exhibiting language of confusion, was rarely observed or reported. Finally, there was no indication in his medical history that he had suffered a closed head injury or any neurological insults that would be consistent with the diagnosis of language of confusion.

Our review of case history information and neuroradiodiagnostic findings also did not provide the information needed to differentiate between aphasia and language of generalized intellectual impairment. For example, sudden onset of his language impairment and the absence of previous neurological or communicative deficits were consistent with an aphasia diagnosis. Alternately, Mr. S.'s history of alcohol abuse was consistent with more generalized brain damage as is often seen in patients exhibiting this language of generalized intellectual impairment. Results of neuroimaging did not resolve these issues, as cortical atrophy and a recent infarction in the left posterior parieto-occipital region were both present.

As mentioned above, Mr. S.'s sudden onset of neurological and language impairment was suggestive of an aphasia diagnosis. In reviewing his BDAE subtest scores, striking differences were apparent in the quality of language produced in response to visual as opposed to auditory stimuli. As aphasic patients typically have equal difficulty on naming tasks regardless of modality of presentation (Goodglass, Barton, & Kaplan, 1968), this was an unexpected finding, and led us to examine the nature of Mr. S.'s visual deficits more closely.

Despite near-normal performance on language tasks that were not visually biased, Mr. S. was markedly impaired on auditory comprehension and naming tasks that required visuolinguistic processing. For example, performance on BDAE auditory comprehension tasks, such as body-part identification, was essentially within normal limits. By contrast, ability to point to objects named, a task requiring visuolinguistic processing, was severely impaired (fortieth percentile; BDAE). Similarly, average performance on BDAE nonvisual naming tasks was at the eightieth percentile, while visual confrontation naming was at the thirty-fifth percentile.

Finally, the discrepancy between the patient's ability to process information through the auditory versus visual modality also was seen on reading comprehension tasks. That is, he performed without error on the BDAE oral spelling subtests, an auditory task. Yet, he performed poorly on word–picture matching tasks.

Mr. S.'s visual impairment resembled a visual agnosia. According to Bauer and Rubens (1985), "the patient with visual agnosia does not respond appropriately to visually presented material even though visual sensory processing, language, and general intellectual functions are preserved at sufficient levels so that their impairment cannot account individually or in combination for the failure to recognize." Especially during initial speech and language testing, when Mr. S. was completely unable to interpret any pictured or printed stimuli, his behaviors were consistent with those seen in this syndrome. Even when the clinician provided the label for an object, Mr. S. was adamant that the clinician was providing the wrong name. Additionally, at the time of follow-up testing, tactile naming was intact while visual naming was impaired, which is characteristic of this disorder.

In contrast to severe deficits on visual linguistic tasks, Mr. S.'s ability to complete *nonlanguage visual tasks* was only mildly-to-moderately impaired. Specifically, he was able to match objects and pictures, copy geometric shapes, and make figure-ground discriminations. Many of the paraphasias produced by Mr. S. demonstrated considerable semantic knowledge regarding target objects, such as when he called a sink a "water-keeper." These findings were originally considered to be inconsistent with a diagnosis of visual agnosia. However, the role of visual perception and recognition in visual agnosia has been disputed in the literature. Bauer and Rubens (1985) suggest that the clinical picture of agnosia typically includes ability to draw or match visually presented pictures of misnamed items. Others, such as Lhermitte and Beauvois (1973), accept the classic view that a diagnosis of visual agnosia excludes individuals that exhibit essentially normal recognition and perception of misnamed objects. The behavioral characteristics that distinguish visual agnosia from other visual-verbal disconnection syndromes are often unclear (Benson, 1979; Poeck, 1984).

In extreme cases where there is a complete visual-verbal disconnection, the label of "optic aphasia" has been applied. Given the outstanding modality specific-language problem exhibited by Mr. S., this diagnosis was reasonable. Optic aphasia was first introduced by Freund (1888) in a report of a case exhibiting a left parieto-occipital area tumor. This patient exhibited a deficit in visual confrontation naming in the context of normal or near normal visual perception. It was hypothesized that a disconnection between the right occipital region and the left language areas accounted for this deficit. Freund's patient also demonstrated aphasia and a right homonymous hemianopsia. Bauer and Rubens (1985) defined "optic aphasia" as a disorder in which "patients are unable to name visually presented objects and yet are able to show that they recognize the object either by indicating its use or by pointing to it when it is named" (p. 203). As was the case for Mr. S., tactile and auditory naming are preserved in this syndrome. At the time of follow-up testing, Mr. S. demonstrated only mildly reduced performance on all visual tasks with the exception of visuolinguistic tasks, which remained severely compromised. Therefore, a disconnection between left hemisphere language areas and right hemisphere occipital (visual) areas, as has been hypothesized in optic aphasia, adequately accounted for Mr. S.'s deficits.

The primary distinction between visual agnosia and optic aphasia is that the agnosias are a disturbance of recognition while optic aphasia is a modality-specific language disorder. Both syndromes are, in fact, relatively rare. Moreover, the distinctions between these two disorders may actually be a matter of severity rather than true qualitative differences (Bauer & Rubens, 1985). Some authors do not distinguish optic aphasia and visual agnosia (Benson, 1979).

There have been several recent reports of visual-verbal disconnection syndromes in the literature. Lhermitte and Beauvois (1973), for example, provide a case report of a patient who experienced an ischemic accident in the left posterior cerebral artery who exhibited normal language except for naming objects in the visual modality, alexia without agraphia, and essentially normal visual perception and recognition. They concluded that their patient demonstrated the same disorder as Freund's case, but preferred the term "visual-speech disconnexion." Poeck (1984) similarly presented a report of a patient who demonstrated "optic anomia" following an ischemic infarction of the left posterior cerebral artery. Characteristics of generally adequate language skills, right homonymous hemianopsia, alexia, and a striking inability to perform visual naming tasks were reported. Additionally, Gil, Pluchon, Toullat, et al. (1985) described a case of "optic aphasia" characterized by a deficit in naming visually presented objects, and alexia with no disturbance of visual perception. Finally, Pena-Casanova, Roig-Rovira, Bermudez, and Tolosa-Sarro (1985) described a patient "without aphasia" who demonstrated alexia without agraphia, color agnosia, and an inability to name objects and pictures in the context of only mild visual perceptual deficits. The site of lesion in this case was the left temporo-occipital area, following a posterior cerebral artery CVA. A visual–verbal disconnection was again hypothesized to account for these deficits.

CONCLUSION

After analyzing Mr. S.'s test results and reviewing the available literature, we concluded that he exhibited a visual–verbal disconnection syndrome as a result of a posterior cerebral artery infarction. There was no obvious explanation for why his confusion persisted for a significantly longer period than is generally reported in the literature. However, at three months post-onset, his confusional state had essentially resolved and what remained was essentially normal or only minimally impaired language skills *except for severe alexia and an almost complete inability to name visually presented objects and pictures.* This occurred in the presence of only mild visual perceptual impairments. Mr. S.'s etiology of posterior cerebral artery CVA and his associated right homonymous hemianopsia, agitation, and confusion were also consistent with the clinical picture described in the literature (Brazis, Masdeu, & Biller, 1985).

In reviewing our initial diagnostic question, Mr. S. did not demonstrate a true aphasia; his deficit was limited to a single (visual) modality, and he did not exhibit language of confusion or language secondary to generalized intellectual impairment. Rather, he demonstrated an apparent disconnection between left hemisphere language areas and right hemisphere visual areas, so that visual information was recognized and appreciated, but it could not be utilized during completion of linguistic tasks. In the final analysis, time and additional observation and testing will determine whether this diagnosis should be expanded or further modified in the future.

REFERENCES

Bauer, R., & Rubens, A. (1985). Agnosia. In K. Heilman & E. Valenstein (Eds.), *Clinical neuropsychology* (2nd ed.). New York: Oxford University Press.

Benson, D.F. (1979). *Aphasia, alexia and agraphia.* New York: Churchill Livingstone.

Brazis, P., Masdeu, J., & Biller, J. (1985). *Localization in clinical neurology.* Boston: Little, Brown and Company.

Devinsky, O., Bear, D., & Volpe, B. (1988). Confusional states following posterior cerebral artery infarction. *Archives of Neurology, 45,* 160-163.

Freund, C. (1888). Ueber optische aphasie and seelenblindheit. *Archiv Fur Psychiatrie und Nervenkrankheiten (Berlin), 20,* 276-297 and 371-416.

Frostig, M. (1966). *Developmental test of visual perception.* Palo Alto, CA: Consulting Psychologists Press.

Gil, R., Pluchon, C., Toullat, G., Micheneau, D., Rogez, R., & Lefevre, J. (1985). Disconnexion visuo-verbale (aphasie optique) pour les objets less images, les couleurs et les visages avec alexie "abstractive." *Neuropsychologia, 23,* 333-349.

Goodglass, H., Barton, M., & Kaplan, E. (1968). Sensory modality and object-naming in aphasics. *Journal of Speech and Hearing Research, 11,* 488-496.

Goodglass, H., & Kaplan, E. (1983). *The assessment of aphasia and related disorders* (2nd ed.). Philadelphia: Lea and Febiger.

Lhermitte, F., & Beauvois, M. (1973). A visual-speech disconnexion syndrome: Report of a case with optic aphasia, agnosic alexia, and colour agnosia. *Brain, 96,* 695-714.

Pena-Casanova, J., Roig-Rovira, T., Bermudez, A., & Tolosa-Sarro, E. (1985). Optic aphasia, optic apraxia, and loss of dreaming. *Brain and Language, 26,* 63-71.

Poeck, K. (1984). Neuropsychological demonstration of splenial interhemispheric disconnection in a case of "optic anomia." *Neuropsychologia, 22,* 707-713.

Wechsler, D. (1945). *Wechsler memory scale.* New York: The Psychological Corporation.

Wertz, R. (1985). Neuropathologies of speech and language: An introduction to patient management. In D. Johns (Ed.), *Clinical management of neurogenic communicative disorders* (2nd ed.). Boston: Little, Brown and Company.

SECTION V

ATYPICAL SPEECH
PROBLEMS
COMPLICATING
THE CLASSIFICATION
OF APHASIA

CHAPTER 12

JOHN C. ROSENBEK
ROSS LEVINE
JO ANNE ROBBINS

WHEN THE ATYPICAL
IS REALLY TYPICAL

A neurology resident sent a consult to the Audiology and Speech Pathology service that said: "63 y-o-male with mild aphasia after left MCA stroke." This consult was received five days after the patient's episode. We read the chart, met the patient, and began informal and then formal speech–language assessment. The patient also served as an experimental subject in a research project to measure the effects of stroke on swallowing.

BRIEF HISTORY

This 63-year-old, right-handed man had graduated from high school, served in the army, and then returned to his hometown to begin life as a chef at a variety of restaurants and lodges. He was described as "a good cook and entertainer who gave parties and had many friends." Alcohol and substance abuse were not reported, and in fact the patient was described as "a virtual teetotaler." His medical history included severe urethral stricture since catheter insertion following hernia repair 19 years previously, exogenous obesity, hypertension, and diabetes mellitus. Prior neurological illness, including transient ischemic attacks, had never been reported.

On the day of his episode, he was described as being in his usual state of health until he collapsed while walking. His local physician noted aphasia, right-sided weakness, and high blood pressure. He was immediately transferred to the Madison Veterans Administration Hospital.

NEUROLOGICAL EXAMINATION

On initial examination performed five hours after onset of neurological symptomatology, the patient was described as being lethargic and unable to speak or consistently comply with the requirements of the examination. Abnormal findings included right-sided neglect, right flaccid hemiplegia, arm greater than legs, right homonymous hemianopsia, right facial weakness, and deviation of tongue to the right. The initial diagnosis was that this patient had a thrombotic left middle cerebral artery (MCA) stroke syndrome. Serial clinical examinations confirmed the original description and served to reenforce the MCA stroke diagnosis.

SPEECH–LANGUAGE EXAMINATION

Prior to a formal examination 9 and 10 days after the onset, the patient was seen for several bedside visits. His illness and the press of other medical tests and procedures decreed that these visits be brief and that conclusions based on them be impressionistic and tentative.

For the formal examination, the unpublished Mayo Clinic Aphasia Examination was used to sample reading, writing, listening, and aspects of verbal expression including naming, proverb explanation, imitation, cloze, and production of serials. Naming was also tested with the Boston Naming Test (Kaplan, Goodglass, & Weintraub, 1983). The Reading Comprehension Battery for Aphasia (RCBA) (LaPointe & Horner, 1979), provided further data on reading. Oral motor performance was tested with a standard speech sample and an oral–peripheral examination.

The following description is based on both informal and formal testing. It is divided by modality.

AUDITORY COMPREHENSION

At four days post-onset the patient was reported by ward staff to be understanding everything. Our assessment, beginning on day five, confirmed that he did respond appropriately but inconsistently to predictable social exchanges and some typical hospital ward conversations and interactions. By day nine, it was determined formally that he could point to single words when named (12/12 correct), could follow some simple, one-step commands involving body parts and objects in the room (8/12 correct), and had more difficulty with more complex commands (3/8 correct). Ability to understand and recall the details of a paragraph were not tested until long after the patient's diagnosis was established.

READING COMPREHENSION

Reading was originally difficult to test because of his lethargy and visual field deficit. Informally, we were able to position large print, single words appropriately in his visual field and demonstrate that he could read them (5/5 correct). Later we attempted the RCBA (LaPointe & Horner, 1979). He rejected the test after scoring 16/20 on the first two subtests. It was not until after his diagnosis was established that we could test reading more completely.

WRITING

Writing was profoundly impaired. Even by day 10, he could not consistently copy even simple letters, and he was totally incapable of writing letters, words, or sentences from dictation. He could spontaneously write his first name but not his last. He could not copy nor draw geometric forms. Considerable diagnostic therapy convinced us that his writing deficits were influenced by, but were not primarily the result of, his visual involvement and/or his lethargy. A sample of his copying (A) and an attempt at his name (B), completed on day 10 appear in Figure 12-1.

VERBAL EXPRESSION

SPONTANEOUS SPEECH

Variability was the hallmark of this patient's verbal expression. Sometimes he was lethargic and had to be prodded to respond even with single words. Even when he did not need to be prodded he often responded with only one or two words. On the other hand, he sometimes produced complete utterances, such as "I have two nieces and a nephew." Such utterances, however, were infrequent, and the same ones seldom appeared twice. Far more frequently he would briefly try to respond then stop and explain, "I can't say it," or he would simply not respond. Literal and verbal paraphasias were rare.

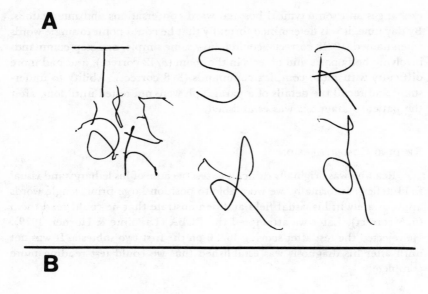

Figure 12-1. Examples of patient's attempt to (A) copy and (B) write his name taken from testing on day 10.

IMITATION

He correctly repeated only 1 of 10 sentences, but was nearly accurate on all 10. His only errors were to omit one or more words from each. For example, he said "What time will bus pick you up?" for "What time will *the* bus pick you up?"

NAMING

Naming was seriously impaired. He scored a 3 on the Boston Naming Test (Kaplan, Goodglass, & Weintraub, 1983). On those few occasions when he would attempt to name, he made within-class word substitutions, which he would then reject as wrong. Usually if the name was not immediately forthcoming he would merely say, "I don't know." Phonemic cues were not helpful.

ORAL MOTOR PERFORMANCE

The patient had a trace of right-sided facial and lingual weakness. His connected speech, limited as it was, was mildly imprecise. Other symptoms were sound and syllable repetitions, reduced loudness and pitch changes, and hypophonia. In addition, he had irregular, inappropriate but mild changes in rate, stress, and rhythm, which gave his speech an ataxic quality.

SWALLOWING EVALUATION

Videofluoroscopic recordings were used to examine oropharyngeal function during swallowing 21 days post-onset. Testing was delayed until this time because of experimental protocol restrictions and because the patient gave no sign of significant dysphagia. Mean duration of the oral stage of swallowing was abnormally long (3.8 seconds). Mean duration of the pharyngeal stage was normal (1.0 seconds). The oral phase of swallowing was characterized by delayed initiation, repetitive lingual motions, palatal coating, and residue on the tongue dorsum. Coating and residue are usually indicative of reduced range of lingual motion and/or weakness. Triggering of the swallow response was delayed for all swallows. Although vallecular stasis was consistently evinced prior to pharyngeal activity, the pharyngeal phase appeared relatively normal once it was initiated.

INITIAL IMPRESSIONS

The patient's aphasia was characterized by severe deficits in writing and naming, and by less severe deficits in auditory and reading comprehension and imitation. Verbal expression was highly variable and seemed to reflect deficits in attention and alertness, as well as aphasia. He was also mildly to moderately dysarthric and mildly dysphagic. He did not have a significant number of paraphasias, nor did he have apraxia of speech.

THE DIFFICULTY

Patients sometimes — perhaps oftentimes — do not turn out to have what professionals think they have. No member of the health care team has a monopoly on making these mistaken diagnoses. All professionals risk being fooled, especially by acutely ill patients. The threats to positive diagnosis accumulate, however, for team members; this includes aphasiologists who, as consultants, not only receive a consult, but also the impressions of the referral source. Perhaps most handicapping of all to the aphasiologist's clear perception is the traditional notion that aphasia, the left MCA and Broca's area, Wernicke's area, and the arcuate fasciculus are inextricably linked.

All members of the team recognized that this patient's aphasia was peculiar. The Speech Pathology consultant wrote, for example, that there was a "minor lobe" quality about his writing. Nonetheless, calling the communication deficit aphasia seemed appropriate. Nor did the ward team have trouble with the notion that the MCA was implicated, even though the aphasia was not typical of those resulting from cortical lesions of Broca's area, Wernicke's area, or the arcuate fasciculus. The speech pathologist, impressed as much by the hypophonic, monotonous, and dyscoordinated speech as by the language findings, suggested that the lesion might involve the basal ganglia, thereby implicating striate branches of the MCA. A consulting Stroke Service neurologist initially suggested a trunk occlusion of the left MCA leading to both basal ganglia and cortical lesions.

The lateral lenticulostriate branches of the MCA nourish the internal capsule, and portions of the basal ganglia and thalamus. Research (Damasio, Damasio, Rizzo, Varney, & Gersh, 1982) has described aphasia and dysarthria following involvement of these branches. Therefore, implicating the MCA seemed a logical conclusion. A cranial computed tomographic (CCT) scan done on day two was unremarkable.

THE ANSWER

A CCT scan done on day 11 finally brought this patient's problem into focus for our rehabilitation team. The formal CCT scan interpretation suggested "evidence of infarction in distribution of left posterior cerebral artery (PCA) involving parieto-occipital cortex, mesial temporal cortex, posterior internal capsule, and thalamus." Selected slices from that scan appear in Figure 12-2. All members of the rehabilitation and ward teams began shamefacedly saying, "Of course. We knew something wasn't quite right."

THE POSTERIOR CEREBRAL ARTERY AND ITS SYNDROMES

If our experience is typical, clinical aphasiologists are most likely to think of the PCA when a patient has a pure, or relatively pure, alexia. Aphasiologists are less likely to think of the PCA when a patient presents

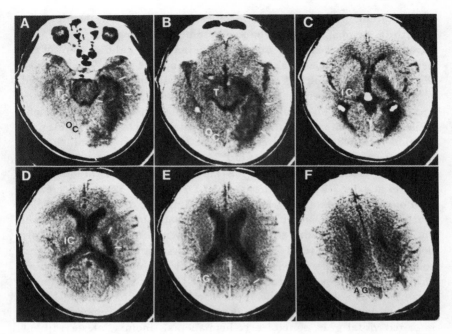

Figure 12-2. CCT scan taken on this 63-year-old patient 11 days post-onset of a PCA territory stroke. A section through the mid-brain (A) reveals mesial temporal (TC) and occipital (OC) cortical infarction. A slightly higher section through the mid-brain and third ventricle (B) shows extension of the infarction into the thalamus (T). Sections through the basal ganglia (C,D) reveals posterior internal capsular (IC) infarction, while a section through the body of the lateral ventricles (E) and superior to the ventricles (F) show infarction of the angular gyrus (AG). (Courtesy of Dr. R. Levine).

with other speech–language signs and symptoms. A review of the PCA distribution, of this patient and of the clinical literature, however, serves as a gentle reminder of this artery's importance to speech, language, and cognitive abilities.

Cortical branches of the PCA serve the occipital cortex, mesial and inferior temporal cortex, and the border zone between occipital and parietal cortices, often including the angular gyrus. Deep perforating branches supply, in a variable fashion, portions of the thalamus, internal capsule, and basal ganglia.

The dangers of diagnostic correlations of vascularity and behavior, especially speech, language, and cognitive behaviors, are well recognized (Kertesz, 1983). It can be hypothesized, however, that our patient's signs and symptoms are related to involvement of specific branches of the PCA. The patient's lethargy and general lack of attention to the environment may have resulted from involvment of the mesencephalic artery. The hemiparesis, dysarthria, dysphagia, and perhaps even some of the language deficit, may have resulted from involvement of the posterior choroidal branch or of the perforating subcortical branches (the thalamoperforates). The language disturbance, including the poor writing and naming, may have resulted primarily from involvement of the posterior temporal branch or the parieto-occipital branch. The visual loss probably resulted from either involvement of the calcarine branch or the parieto-occipital branch. The hemineglect probably resulted from involvement of the parieto-occipital branch.

The usual presenting features of PCA territory infarctions are described by Kinkel, Newman, and Jacobs (1984) and involve visual field loss on the opposite side (76.5%), hemiparesis (47.1%), confusion (32.4%), decreased level of consciousness (14.7%), and speech–language disturbance (8.8%). Our patient is similar to at least 2 of the 34 patients described by Kinkel and colleagues, suggesting that his deficits, albeit infrequent, are certainly not unique and are lawfully related to the PCA's distribution. Kinkel's and colleague's (1984) reference can serve as a guide to the clinical recognition of PCA patients. Another useful reference is Caplan's (1980) description of various rostral brainstem and hemispheric effects of basilar artery, including PCA, involvement. These include disorders of ocular movement, such as impaired visual gaze, somnolence, hemianopia, anomia, alexia without agraphia, and a "temporary Korsakoff-like amnestic syndrome."

Improving Our Insight

Debate about classification in aphasia is increasingly more frequent and more heated. Darley (1982) wrote a long denial of the adjective's (conduction, transcortical motor, Broca's, and Wernicke's) place in the classification of aphasia. Schwartz (1984) and Caramazza (1984) both believe in types of aphasia, but deny the usefulness of existing classification systems. Schwartz says that the polytypic structure of existing systems, in which members of a group need not share any single feature or pattern of features, makes their use in neurolinguistic research impossible. Caramazza says group research with existing types "is not theoretically defensible."

When debate increases, so do efforts to resolve it. Caramazza's solution is exhaustive testing of single patients. A companion strategy may be to devise different classification systems. Poeck (1983) proposes a system based on the brain's vascularization. He even suggests that the classical syndromes of aphasia "are, to a large extent, artifacts produced by vascularization of the language area" (p. 84).

Our case was an excellent test of the vascularization approach. We, however, appreciated this more on the eleventh day after the stroke than before it. Our patient's symptoms were apparently the predictable result of a specific pattern of PCA involvement. Presumably, different clusters of signs and symptoms result from other patterns of PCA involvement.

REFERENCES

Caplan, L.R. (1980). "Top of the basilar" syndrome. *Neurology, 30*, 72-79.

Caramazza, A. (1984). The logic of neuropsychological research and the problem of patient classification in aphasia. *Brain and Language, 21*, 9-20.

Damasio, A.R., Damasio, H., Rizzo, M., Varney, N., & Gersh, F. (1982). Aphasia with nonhemorrhagic lesions in the basal ganglia and internal capsule. *Archives of Neurology, 39*, 15-20.

Darley, F.L. (1982). *Aphasia*. Philadelphia: Saunders.

Kaplan, E., Goodglass, H., & Weintraub, S. (1983). *Boston naming test*. Philadelphia: Lea and Febiger.

Kertesz, A. (1983). *Localization in neuropsychology*. New York: Academic Press.

Kinkel, W.R., Newman, R.P., & Jacobs, L. (1984). Posterior cerebral artery branch occlusions: CT and anatomic considerations. In R. Berguer & R.B. Bauer (Eds.), *Vertebrobasilar arterial occlusive disease* (pp. 117-133). New York: Raven Press.

LaPointe, L.L., & Horner, J. (1979). *Reading comprehension battery for aphasia*. Tigard, OR: C.C. Publications.

Poeck, K. (1983). What do we mean by "aphasic syndromes?" A neurologists' view. *Brain and Language, 20*, 79-89.

Schwartz, M.F. (1984). What the classical aphasia categories can't do for us, and why. *Brain and Language, 21*, 3-8.

CHAPTER 13

THOMAS E. PRESCOTT

A CASE OF TRANSCORTICAL SENSORY APHASIA?

A request for speech–language consultation was received for Mr. S. from the medical center intensive care unit. The request stated, "Patient status post left cerebrovascular accident with aphasia, needs rehabilitation." Informal assessment on the same day the consult was received showed "decreased auditory comprehension and decreased reading comprehension." The patient was scheduled for more formalized speech and language assessment.

HISTORY

Mr. S. was a 57-year-old insurance adjuster, married and the father of one grown child. He apparently had no speech–language difficulties prior to a recent hospital admission for an increased problem with diabetes mellitus. He was reported to be an insulin-dependent diabetic with poor glucose control secondary "to chronic renal failure neuropathy."

On the day prior to his planned hospital discharge, Mr. S. experienced a left hemorrhagic bleed into the left basal ganglia resulting in right hemiparesis and aphasia. The stroke was described as "major, resulting in severe disability."

Shortly after the stroke, chart notes described Mr. S. as an alert male, unable to provide the date, unreliable in providing information, and sometimes unable to follow commands. Neurology chart notes described a patient who was alert and cooperative when he understood the issue or the request. He had a flaccid right arm and 2/5 proximal right leg strength.

Within days following his stroke, Mr. S. was noted to be aspirating his oral food intake. His aspiration problems were confirmed by radiological study. Because he experienced repeated episodes of aspiration pneumonia, a gastrostomy tube was inserted.

Speech and Language Status

Initial formal evaluation of Mr. S. specific to his speech and language capabilities was initiated three days after the left cerebrovascular accident. We discontinued attempts to administer the Boston Diagnostic Aphasia Examination (Goodglass & Kaplan, 1983) because the patient, at that time, was experiencing multiple life-threatening events. At one month post-onset, however, testing was completed using the Porch Index of Communicative Abilities (PICA) (Porch, 1981). The results are shown in Table 13-1, and subsequently will be compared to the results at five months post-onset.

These PICA results at one month post-onset described a patient with a severe communication deficit, who was predicted to reach the twenty-third percentile overall at six months post-onset. Auditory processing was severely compromised for objects named by the examiner (tenth percentile) and for descriptive functions of the object (twelfth percentile). He produced only unintelligible utterances when attempting to name objects (first percentile). Occasionally he rejected attempts at the task. When asked to repeat the names of objects, Mr. S. demonstrated variability in his response pattern. He produced one correct but delayed repetition, and one correct response, following repetition of the stimulus. In addition to the responses he produced correctly, Mr. S. produced a number of inaccurate but intelligible imitative responses. The remainder of his responses, however, remained unintelligible. Writing was nonfunctional, but he could read simple words for comprehension. Of particular interest was his fluent word-for-word, accurate repetition of longer complex sentence units (Mayo Clinic Apraxia Battery sentences). Mr. S. was tentatively classified at this point in time as exhibiting transcortical sensory aphasia (even though the profile was not ideal), because of his unique ability to correctly repeat long sentence units in the face of poor auditory comprehension.

Speech and Language Treatment Outcome

Mr. S. was enrolled in an individual speech–language treatment program scheduled for five times a week. In actuality, treatment was intermittent due to his recurring medical problems. These problems included difficulties with the above mentioned insulin regulation, aspiration pneumonia, renal malfunctions, and problems associated with his gastric tube which required corrective surgery. A problem-oriented list for Mr. S. identified 16 different areas requiring medical intervention.

Mr. S. was transferred to the medical center nursing home care unit but continued to experience a wide range of medical problems which prevented discharge to his home. Occasionally he was readmitted to the hospital for needed medical treatment.

Despite his recurrent medical problem, Mr. S. demonstrated improvement in his speech–language skills. Five months after his onset of CVA he achieved the levels on the PICA as shown in Table 13-1.

Contrasted with his performance at one month post-onset, Mr. S.'s performance at five months had exceeded the level predicted for him based on his first PICA scores. He could now repeat single words with complete accuracy. His naming abilities had improved considerably from mostly unintelligible utterances to mostly accurate, rather slow naming with only occasional errors. Sentence completion had improved significantly, as had descriptions of object functions. Repetition of single words was now 90 percent accurate, and imitation of longer utterances remained intact.

DISCUSSION

Classification of the aphasia exhibited by Mr. S. was of interest, particularly in view of his initially poor ability to repeat single words, but intact ability to repeat long sentences (e.g., "The shipwreck washed up on the shore."). Although this pattern seemed atypical, we asked if Mr. S. exhibited what several writers have labeled as transcortical sensory aphasia. Goodglass and Kaplan (1972) state the following regarding transcortical sensory aphasia:

TABLE 13-1.
Mr. S.'s percentile scores on the PICA.

Test	One Month Post-onset	Five Months Post-onset
Overall	14	40
Writing	5	57
Copying	15	22
Reading	12	30
Pantomime	15	20
Verbal	25	54
Auditory	11	25
Visual	11	14

The typical patient with this disorder does not initiate speech on his own. When addressed, he replies with well articulated, but irrelevant paraphasia which may include both actual English words and neologisms. He is totally unable to name to confrontation but usually offers grossly irrelevant responses when so stimulated. These patients often echo the examiner's words instead of replying. However their ability to repeat is not limited to echoing, as they may, on request, listen to and repeat back correctly sentences of considerable length and complexity. (p. 72)

Other writers concur with this description of transcortical sensory aphasia, including Davis (1983), Brown (1972), Geschwind, Quadfasel, and Segarra (1968), and Kertesz (1979). With the exception of the absence of the echoic behaviors, Mr. S. appeared to demonstrate transcortical sensory aphasia. Mr. S.'s most noticeable deficits were a severe auditory processing disorder and naming difficulty. Surprisingly, although he was poor at repeating single words he was able, without error, to repeat long sentences.

In addition, the locus of the lesion described for this patient appeared consistent with lesion sites previously reported and associated with transcortical sensory aphasia. Mr. S. was reported to have experienced a "left hemorrhagic bleed into the area of the left basal ganglia." Yamadori, Ohira, Seriu, and Ogura (1984) described three patients with lesions of the left basal ganglia. These patients were labeled as having transcortical sensory aphasia with the features listed in Table 13-2. Test results and behavioral observations of Mr. S. indicated that he exhibited fluent speech output, poor naming, and poor auditory comprehension, but preserved capacity for repetition of sentences (although not single words). The fifth characteristic, reading aloud, was not tested, but his reading comprehension was severely impaired. The final characteristic, writing, was profoundly compromised across tasks. In overall comparison, Mr. S. appears to meet several, but not all, of the behaviors associated with transcortical sensory aphasia. Finally, Brown (1972) discussed the importance of distinguishing

---

TABLE 13-2.
Characteristics of hemorrhagic patients with left basal ganglia lesions.

- Fluent paraphasic verbal output
- Anomia that was not facilitated by cueing
- Impaired comprehension of spoken language
- Preserved capacity of repetition
- Preserved ability to read aloud with impaired comprehension of written material
- Agraphia

Adapted from Yamadori, Ohira, Seriu, & Ogura, 1984.

> ... between echolalia at the word and at the phrase level, the former being a common occurrence in sensory aphasia, the latter more specifically associated with transcortical aphasia, isolation syndrome cases and the echolalia of dementia. (p. 73)

These issues raise the possibility of other classifications for Mr. S.'s constellation of symptoms. Kertesz (1979) describes an isolation-of-the-speech-areas syndrome characterized by fluent speech, good repetition, and auditory comprehension difficulty. In addition, echolalia associated with dementia has also been described (Whitaker, 1976).

The precise classification of the patient's aphasia, however, may be more or less important depending upon the aim of the rehabilitation program. In the case of Mr. S., we were faced with the task of trying to improve his functional communication skills. Instead of struggling with a classification, we chose to identify and describe his deficits and to modify those behaviors that prevented good communication. Treatment for Mr. S. consisted primarily of tasks aimed toward improving his auditory processing skills. These included practice in following commands, pointing to pictures, pointing to printed words, and pointing to objects when functions were described. In addition, stimuli presentations were modified (Blanchard & Prescott, 1980; Marshall, 1978; Salvatore, 1975) with pause insertion, reduced presentation rate, use of alerting signals, and so on. Manipulations of the stimuli (e.g., number of stimuli presented, semantic field) also were employed (Marshall, 1978). Practice was conducted on visual matching tasks, imitation of monosyllabic words with bilabial initial consonants, and naming using a sentence completion technique for pictured items. Mr. S. demonstrated improvement, but did not master any of these areas completely. Following five months of treatment utilizing this approach, considerable change and improvement was observed for this patient.

While we were pleased with the improvements in this patient's communicative ability, it may be that the treatment had less to do with recovery than did the natural evolution of the disorder, despite the poor prognosis indicated by his PICA scores. PICA six-month predictions for Mr. S. were exceeded (approximately doubled) at five months post-onset, as noted in Table 13-1. Perhaps PICA scores do not predict recovery well for subcortical lesion patients or do not account for treatment effects. In any case, Mr. S.'s test performance considerably exceeded the PICA predicted level, in spite of his recurrent medical problems. Kertesz (1979) suggests that transcortical sensory aphasia, especially if traumatically caused, is transient, but the etiology of Mr. S.'s aphasia was hemorrhagic. Yamadori and colleagues (1984) suggested that lesions of the basal ganglia, such as they reported, had not previously been reported as resulting in transcortical sensory aphasia.

Variations in deficit from classical descriptions have been suggested by Coslett, Roeltgen, Rothi, and Heilman (1987). These authors indicated the presence of subtypes of transcortical sensory aphasia. McCarthy and Warrington (1987) suggested that repetition skills (memory for lists and sentences) in their transcortical sensory aphasic patients were not facilitated by meaningfulness of the stimuli. These authors hypothesized the existence of a differing short-term memory system in patients with conduction aphasia versus transcortical sensory aphasia. Finally, behaviors and deficits exhibited by patients with subcortical "deep" lesions have been reported. Nine fluent aphasics with deep lesions were described by Basso, Della Sala, and Ferabola (1987). These authors concluded, "a consistent relationship between site of lesion and the pattern of aphasic disturbances could not be established." In contrast, Alexander, Naeser, and Palumbo (1987) concluded from their study of 19 patients with subcortical lesions that different syndromes of aphasic deficit are related to differing lesion loci. These authors stated, "Simple tabulation of lesions as cortical or subcortical, and restricting analysis to lesions of basal ganglia would both have proved inadequate to account for our clinical findings" (p. 961).

The existing literature points out the inadequacy of the clinical data available to us for confident classification of Mr. S.'s aphasia. The need for clinical study and data on a considerably expanded level than was accomplished for Mr. S. is apparent. This need includes more sophistication in lesion localization, as well as more precise description of the patient's communication deficit.

We believe Mr. S. exhibited transcortical sensory aphasia. Our clinical task, however, was not to classify the type of disorder but to try to assist this patient with his communicative abilities. This patient demonstrates two major problems in contemporary aphasiology; variations in profiles of behaviors may result in tentative classifications, and responses to treatment are not always predictable.

REFERENCES

Alexander, M., Naeser, M., & Palumbo, C. (1987). Correlations of subcortical CT lesion sites and aphasia profiles. *Brain, 10*, 961–991.

Basso, H., Della Sala, S., & Ferabola, M. (1987). Aphasia arising from purely deep lesion. *Cortex, 23*, 29–44.

Blanchard, S. & Prescott, T. (1980). The effects of temporal expansion upon comprehension in aphasic adults. *British Journal of Disorders of Communication, 15*, 115–127.

Brown, J.W. (1972). *Aphasia, apraxia and agnosia.* Springfield, IL: Charles C Thomas.

Coslett, H., Roeltgen, D., Rothi, L.J.G., & Heilman, K. (1987). Transcortical sensory aphasia: Evidence of subtypes. *Brain and Language, 32*, 362-378.

Davis, G.A. (1983). *A survey of adult aphasia.* Englewood Cliffs, NJ: Prentice-Hall.

Geschwind, N., Quadfasel, F., & Segarra, J. (1968). Isolation of the speech area. *Neuropsychologia, 6*, 327-340.

Goodglass, H. & Kaplan, E. (1972). *Boston diagnostic aphasia examination.* Philadelphia: Lea & Febiger.

Goodglass, H. & Kaplan, E. (1983). *The assessment of aphasia and related disorders.* Philadelphia: Lea and Febiger.

Kertesz, A. (1979). *Aphasias and associated disorders: Taxonomy localization and recovery.* New York: Grune & Stratton.

Marshall, R. (1978). *Clinician controlled auditory stimulation for aphasic adults.* Tigard, Oregon: C.C. Publications.

McCarthy, R. & Warrington, E. (1987). The double dissociation of short-term memory for lists and sentences: Evidence from aphasia. *Brain, 110*(6), 1545-1563.

Porch, B.E. (1981). *Porch index of communicative ability.* Palo Alto, CA: Consulting Psychologists Press.

Salvatore, A. (1975). *The effects of pause duration on sentence comprehension by aphasic individuals.* Paper presented at the American Speech and Hearing Association Convention, Washington, D.C.

Whitaker, H. (1976). A case of the isolation of the language function. In H. Whitaker & H. Whitaker (Eds.), *Studies in neurolinguistics,* (Vol. 2). New York: Academic Press.

Yamadori, A., Ohira, T., Seriu, M., & Ogura, J. (1984). Transcortical sensory aphasia produced by lesions of the anterior basal ganglia area. *No To Shinkei, 36*, 261-266.

CHAPTER 14

ROBERT T. WERTZ
ELLEN G. BERNSTEIN-ELLIS
JAN A. ROBERTS

A CASE OF CONDUCTION APHASIA OR APHASIA AND APRAXIA OF SPEECH

*D*iagnosis implies a prognosis and indicates how a patient will be managed. For some patients, no appropriate management is available. For others, an efficacious treatment exists. Thus, an accurate diagnosis dictates what a patient's future will be and how that future may be attained. While all patients deserve a diagnosis, some do not receive one. The symptoms they display reside beyond our experience and knowledge, and they create a diagnostic dilemma. These cases are important, because they have something to teach us. Our patient, P.G., is such a case.

CASE HISTORY

P.G., a 64-year-old woman, had completed 16 years of education and was right handed. Two CVAs—one in the right hemisphere parietal area, onset unknown, and one in the left hemisphere frontal-temporol-parietal area, six months before we met—had resulted in mild right hemiparesis and speech and language deficits. She had received one month of language treatment two months after she suffered the left hemisphere CVA. Her clinician reported P.G. displayed "moderately severe aphasia and moderate oral–verbal and nonverbal apraxia of speech." And, "good progress" had been achieved during treatment.

EVALUATION

Six months after the CVA, we saw no oral–nonverbal apraxia, and we were not convinced she displayed apraxia of speech. P.G. performed at the eighty-fourth Overall percentile on the Porch Index of Communicative Ability (PICA) (Porch, 1967), using bilateral norms. As shown in Figure 14-1, Gestural performance was at the eighty-fourth percentile, Verbal performance at the forty-second percentile, and Graphic performance at the ninety-eighth percentile. She did not meet any of the PICA bilateral signs: poorer performance on visual subtests than on auditory subtests, inordinately high verbal performance, and inordinately low graphic performance. In fact, her poor verbal performance is what made her enigmatic. Typically, inordinately low verbal ability coexisting with relatively good gestural and graphic abilities signals the presence of either apraxia of speech and/or dysarthria coexisting with aphasia. Absence of significant respiratory, laryngeal, and articulatory weakness, slowness, or lack of coordination ruled out dysarthria, and the presence of apraxia of speech was debatable.

On the Boston Diagnostic Aphasia Examination (BDAE) (Goodglass & Kaplan, 1983), P.G. profiled, as shown in Figure 14-2, within the range of conduction aphasia. Performance on the Western Aphasia Battery (WAB) (Kertesz, 1982) agreed with the BDAE that she displayed conduction aphasia. Her WAB Aphasia Quotient was 55, and, like the BDAE, it indicated fluent aphasia, relatively good auditory comprehension, and extremely impaired verbal repetition.

We wondered whether P.G. was a bona fide conduction aphasic patient or whether she was a fluent aphasic patient with coexisting apraxia of speech. The criteria that we use to differentiate conduction aphasia from apraxia of speech (Table 14-1) indicated P.G. displayed some of the signs for each disorder. She made sequencing errors, but they were fewer than other types of errors. Her substitutions were only somewhat predictable. Prosody was disrupted, but we were not certain this represented apraxia of speech, aprosodia from the right hemisphere brain damage, or was the result of frequent hesitations and interruptions generated by word-finding difficulty. Generally, she was fluent and grammatical, but there were obvious instances of nonfluency and agrammatism. The left hemisphere infarct was both anterior and posterior, and we did not know how the right parietal damage was influencing her behavior. Its presence was undetected until a CT scan

Porch Index of Communicative Ability

MODALITY RESPONSE SUMMARY

Name P. G Case No. ______

Age 64 Birthdate 7/22/20 Sex F Race CAU Handedness RIGHT (R) USED

Diagnosis BILATERAL CVAs Onset LEFT 4/84, RIGHT UNKNOWN

Date 10/10/84 Overall 12.35 Gestural 13.63 Verbal 8.80 Graphic 13.02

Date ______ Overall ______ Gestural ______ Verbal ______ Graphic ______

Date ______ Overall ______ Gestural ______ Verbal ______ Graphic ______

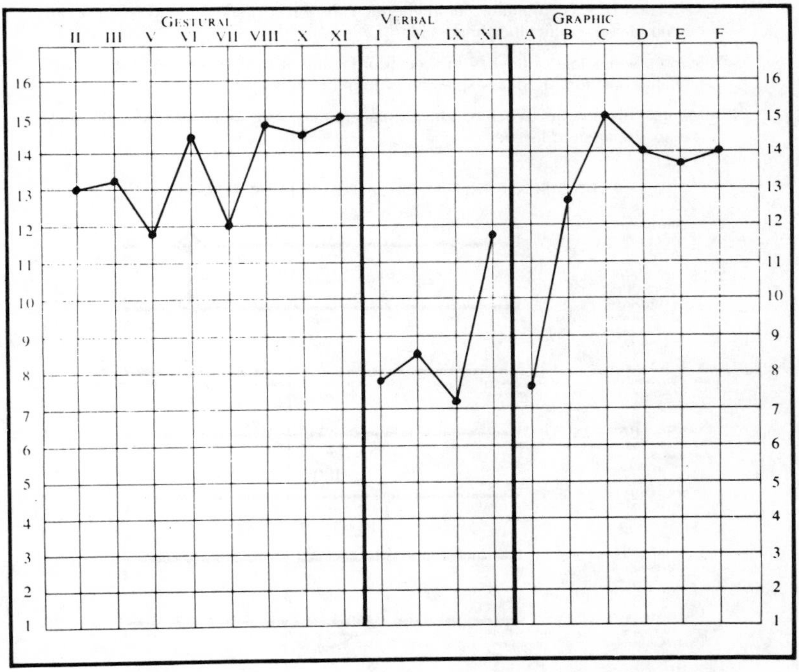

Note ______

Published by
CONSULTING PSYCHOLOGISTS PRESS
577 College Avenue Palo Alto, California

Figure 14-1. PICA Modality Response Summary shows P.G.'s performance at six months post-onset. From Porch, B. (1967). *Porch Index of Communicative Ability*. Palo Alto, CA: Consulting Psychologists Press. Reprinted with permission.

Patient's Name _____ **P. G.** _____   Date of rating _____ **10/15/84** _____
                                           Rated by _____ **R.T.W.** _____

APHASIA SEVERITY RATING SCALE

0. No usable speech or auditory comprehension.

1. All communication is through fragmentary expression; great need for inference, questioning, and guessing by the listener. The range of information that can be exchanged is limited, and the listener carries the burden of communication.

2. Conversation about familiar subjects is possible with help from the listener. There are frequent failures to convey the idea, but patient shares the burden of communication with the examiner.

3. The patient can discuss <u>almost all everyday problems</u> with little or no assistance. Reduction of speech and/or comprehension, however, makes conversation about certain material difficult or impossible.

4. Some obvious loss of fluency in speech or facility of comprehension, without significant limitation on ideas expressed or form of expression.

5. Minimal discernible speech handicaps; patient may have subjective difficulties that are not apparent to listener.

RATING SCALE PROFILE OF SPEECH CHARACTERISTICS

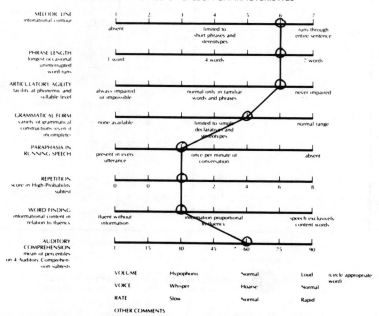

Figure 14-2. BDAE Rating Scale Profile of Speech Characteristics places P.G. within the range of conduction aphasia.

TABLE 14-1.
Criteria for differentiating apraxia of speech from conduction aphasia.

Apraxia of Speech	Conduction Aphasia
Lower proportion of sequencing errors	Higher proportion of sequencing errors
Predictable substitutions	Unpredictable substitutions
Abnormal prosody	Normal prosody
Usually nonfluent	Fluent
Frequently agrammatical	Grammatical
Usually anterior brain damage	Posterior brain damage
Frequently right hemiplegic	Usually not hemiplegic

was done after she sustained the left hemisphere CVA. P.G.'s mild right hemiparesis did not prevent her from writing, gesturing, and eating with her preferred right hand.

A search for the salient signs of apraxia of speech (Wertz, LaPointe, & Rosenbek, 1984) in P.G.'s verbal output contributed additional ambiguity. She displayed some effortful, trial-and-error, groping articulatory movements, and she made numerous attempts to self-correct her errors. Dysprosody was present, but there were periods of normal rhythm, stress, and intonation. Her articulation was not always inconsistent during repeated productions of the same utterance. And, while she had obvious difficulty initiating utterances, it was not always the oral, nonverbal groping movements we typically see in patients who display apraxia of speech. Did she have conduction aphasia or fluent aphasia coexisting with apraxia of speech? Because we could not give P.G. a diagnosis, we decided to see whether her response to treatment would provide one.

RATIONALE

Some years ago, McGinnis (1963) was asked how she knew whether children were aphasic. She indicated that it was easy; if they responded to her treatment, they were aphasic; if they did not, they were not. Rosenbek (1987) has resurrected McGinnis' notion by suggesting a patient's response to a specific treatment may indicate the appropriate diagnosis. For example, in medicine, a positive response to L-dopa may confirm a diagnosis of Parkinson's disease. Of course, it is possible that a specific treatment may be effective for more than one disorder. Nevertheless, we reasoned that if P.G. had apraxia of speech coexisting with fluent aphasia, she would improve when treated with verbal repetition. Many patients with apraxia of speech do (Rosenbek, 1985). Conversely, if she had conduction aphasia, repetition treatment would be ineffective (Simmons, 1983).

P.G. wanted to gain control over her conversation—to reduce the hesitancy, eliminate the interruptions, and improve her word-finding. We were developing a treatment at that time, the Texas Aphasia Contrastive Language Series (TACS) (Roberts & Wertz, 1986), that permitted some patients with aphasia and coexisting apraxia of speech to accomplish most of what P.G. wanted to do. We did not think it would work with a patient who had conduction aphasia, because the initial treatment requires sentence repetition; the most difficult task for this kind of patient.

TREATMENT

TACS requires patients to produce sentences in response to 30 pairs of contrasting pictures. For example, as shown in Figure 14-3, "The door is closed" is contrasted with "The door is open." Treatment progresses through three steps. In Step 1, the clinician produces a sentence for one picture; for example, "The door is open." The patient repeats "The door is open." Then he or she produces a sentence for the other picture; in this example, "The door is closed." Step 2 requires the patient to listen to a sentence describing one picture and then to produce a sentence for the other picture. Step 3 requires the patient to produce a sentence for one picture and then produce a sentence for the other picture. P.G. received 20 one-hour treatment sessions at a rate of one session a day for four weeks.

In Figure 14-4, pretreatment baseline showed Step 3 behavior, spontaneous production of a sentence for each paired picture in a set of 30, was around a score of 9—accurate production after a repetition of instructions— on a modified PICA, 16-point multidimensional scoring system. Criterion

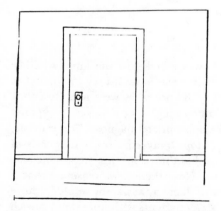
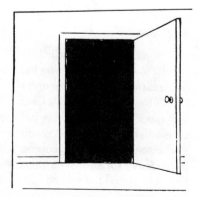

Figure 14-3. Example of TACS paired picture stimuli.

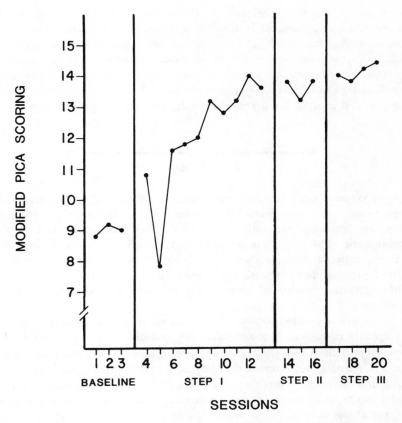

Figure 14-4. P.G.'s pretreatment performance and performance on each step of TACS during treatment.

performance on Step 1, three consecutive sessions at a score of 13 — complete, accurate, but delayed performance — or better, was reached in 10 sessions. Because P.G. was nearing discharge, we did not take time to insert a withdrawal of treatment between steps, even though this is preferable (McReynolds & Kearns, 1983). Criterion was reached on Step 2 after three more sessions, and on Step 3 in four additional sessions.

POST-TREATMENT

Pre- and post-treatment comparison of WAB and PICA performance indicated a 25-point gain in the WAB aphasia quotient, from 55 to 80, and an eight-percentile improvement in the PICA Overall, from the eighty-fourth percentile to the ninety-second. As shown in Figure 14-5, there was a 21-percentile improvement in the PICA Verbal Modality, from the forty-second to the sixty-third. The BDAE was not repeated after treatment, although post-treatment WAB performance classified P.G. as anomic aphasic. Her conversation was quite functional, and she looked forward to her discharge to a Veterans Home in the Napa Valley wine country, where she planned to sit and sip and chat with "all those lonely old men."

DISCUSSION

What was P.G.'s diagnosis before and after treatment? At discharge, her sequencing errors were markedly reduced; substitutions were present but rare, and prosody was mildly abnormal. She was fluent and rarely agrammatic. The mild right hemiparesis persisted. P.G.'s initial diagnosis was conduction aphasia, or fluent aphasia with coexisting apraxia of speech. After treatment, her diagnosis was anomic aphasia, or mild fluent aphasia with coexisting apraxia of speech. We had not resolved the diagnostic dilemma.

P.G. had responded positively to a treatment we believed was appropriate for apraxia of speech. It took a while, 10 sessions, to get her through the repetition on Step 1 of TACS. Was this the result of a petulant conduction aphasia resisting a treatment that required repetition, or was it the slow reduction of apraxic errors that may occur when treating apraxia of speech with repetition? We suspect it was the former. During the contrasting picture treatment, we did not see the oral, nonverbal posturing—starts, stops, and reattempts—and inconsistent articulatory errors typical of the patient who suffers apraxia of speech. Prosody remained mildly disrupted, but this may result from the right hemisphere lesion.

Others (Shewan & Bandur, 1986) have treated conduction aphasia with repetition tasks. Their purpose was not to improve repetition, but to provide a transition to improved spontaneous speech. Sullivan, Fisher, and Marshall (1986) utilized oral reading to treat conduction aphasia and found that it reduced literal and verbal paraphasias, and improved oral sentence reading and single word and low probability sentence repetition. Peach (1987) employed repetition to treat what may be a short-term memory deficit in conduction aphasia. His patient showed gains on post-treatment repetition, naming, and spontaneous speech measures.

So, it appears conduction aphasia may respond to a variety of treatments, including those that require repetition. Does that mean that P.G.'s initial diagnosis should have been conduction aphasia? Not necessarily, but we suspect so. In the context of TACS treatment, the signs that signify

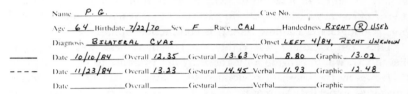

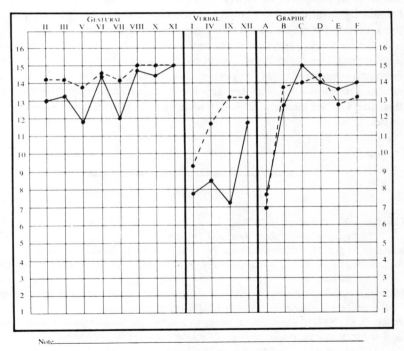

Figure 14-5. P.G.'s pre- and post-treatment performance on the PICA. From Porch, B. (1967). *Porch Index of Communicative Ability.* Palo Alto, CA: Consulting Psychologists Press. Reprinted with permission.

apraxia of speech—effortful, trial-and-error, groping articulatory movements, and attempts at self-correction; dysprosody unrelieved by extended periods of normal rhythm, stress and intonation; articulatory inconsistency on repeated productions of the same utterances; and obvious difficulty initiating utterances—were not observed. Those that indicate conduction aphasia—a high proportion of sequencing errors; unpredictable substitutions; fluent, grammatical speech—were evident. Moreover, repetition difficulty on Step 1 of TACS yielded slowly and was disproportionately impaired in relation to P.G.'s good auditory comprehension and her level of fluency in nonrepetitive parts of the treatment. That, to us and others (Goodglass & Kaplan, 1983), is conduction aphasia.

Thus, our rationale was right, but our hypothesis was wrong. We believed P.G. would provide a diagnosis by her response to treatment. She did. However, the way she responded to treatment did not provide the diagnosis we expected. Moreover, we wonder how often creating the correct context by administering L-dopa to a Parkinson's-like patient may permit the salient signs of pseudobulbar palsy to emerge.

Patients who present a diagnostic dilemma have something to teach us. Our experience with P.G. suggests diagnostic therapy may provide a diagnosis when traditional appraisal fails. Asking what a patient can tell us about diagnosis by his or her response to treatment may yield a surprise. But, this kind of amazement is one of the joys in the work we have elected to do.

REFERENCES

Goodglass, H., & Kaplan, E. (1983). *The assessment of aphasia and related disorders* (2nd ed.). Philadelphia: Lea and Febiger.

Kertesz, A. (1982). *Western aphasia battery*. New York: Grune & Stratton.

McGinnis, M.E. (1963). *Aphasic children*. Washington, DC: Alexander Graham Bell Association.

McReynolds, L.V., & Kearns, K.P. (1983). *Single-subject experimental designs in communicative disorders*. Baltimore: University Park Press.

Peach, R.K. (1987). A short-term memory treatment approach to the repetition deficit in conduction aphasia. In R.H. Brookshire (Ed.), *Clinical aphasiology, volume 17* (pp. 35–45). Minneapolis: BRK Publishers.

Porch, B.E. (1967). *The Porch index of communicative ability*. Palo Alto, CA: Consulting Psychologists Press.

Roberts, J.A., & Wertz, R.T. (1986). A contrastive-language treatment for aphasic adults. In R.H. Brookshire (Ed.), *Clinical aphasiology, volume 16* (pp. 207–212). Minneapolis: BRK Publishers.

Rosenbek, J.C. (1985). Treating apraxia of speech. In D.F. Johns (Ed.), *Clinical management of neurogenic communication disorders*, (2nd ed.). (pp. 267-312). Boston: Little, Brown and Company.

Rosenbek, J.C. (1987, February). *Brain-behavior relationships relevant in aphasia rehabilitation*. Paper presented to the conference on The Aphasic Adult: A Management Approach, Long Beach, California.

Shewan, C.M., & Bandur, D.L. (1986). *Treatment of aphasia: A language oriented approach*. San Diego: College-Hill Press.

Simmons, N.N. (1983). Treatment of conduction aphasia. In W.H. Perkins (Ed.), *Language handicaps in adults* (pp. 45-55). New York: Thieme-Stratton.

Sullivan, M.P., Fisher, B., & Marshall, R.C. (1986). Treating the repetition deficit in conduction aphasia. In R.H. Brookshire (Ed.), *Clinical aphasiology, volume 16* (pp. 172-180). Minneapolis: BRK Publishers.

Wertz, R.T., LaPointe, L.L., & Rosenbek, J.C. (1984). *Apraxia of speech in adults: The disorder and its management*. Orlando, FL: Grune & Stratton.

SECTION VI

**DIAGNOSTIC AND
MANAGEMENT
STRATEGIES FOR
DYSTONIC AND
DYSARTHRIC PATIENTS**

CHAPTER 15

CHRISTY L. LUDLOW
SUSAN E. SEDORY
MIHOKO FUJITA

INSPIRATORY SPEECH WITH RESPIRATORY DYSTONIA

F.C., a 61-year-old woman, was referred in December, 1986, with a diagnosis of spasmodic dysphonia of one year duration. The referring physician's office records reported a history atypical of spasmodic dysphonia. According to his records, F.C. had hoarseness of many years duration, which had been increasing when seen in May, 1984. The physician noted that F.C.'s hoarseness was associated with frequent use of topical steroids inhaled through the larynx. Indirect laryngoscopy in 1984 revealed polypoid thickening and vocal nodules in the mid-third of each fold. The patient was put on voice rest, advised to discontinue inhalants, and referred for voice therapy. She terminated voice therapy after two visits. At that time, she also had dysphagia, and reported that hot food was irritating to swallow. A barium swallow indicated "a mild neuromuscular dysfunction."

In November, 1985, she returned with deteriorating voice, increased vocal fold polyps, and shortness of breath. Vocal fold stripping was performed in December, 1985. The patient had a breathy voice one month after surgery, and voice therapy was initiated. After six months of voice therapy, no voice improvement was noted, although the vocal polyps had not recurred. Gelfoam injections were recommended, but the patient declined. In August,

1986, she was diagnosed as having spasmodic dysphonia, and was placed on a trial of propanolol, which was discontinued because of side effects.

INITIAL EXAMINATION

When first seen by us in December, 1986, F.C. complained of shortness of breath, a feeling of tightness in her ribs, and difficulty breathing when in certain postures, such as sitting in a car. She had severe asthma for which she had used many inhalants over the last 10 years, including Proventil, Venceril, Ventolin, and Aerobid. She underwent three to four treatments per year with large dosages of Prednisone, and had frequent asthmatic attacks with one hospitalization for respiratory failure. She was also taking Zantec for gastric reflux.

She consistently produced speech on inspiration, had severe dyspnea, short breath groups, and a breathy raspy quality. Her vocal quality was improved when directed to speak on expiration, but she was unable to maintain expiratory speech for more than one sentence.

Oral peripheral examination for isometric strength and speed of rapid alternating movements of the tongue, lips, and jaw was within normal limits. Under controlled speech testing conditions using a stimulus tape, her conversational speech was improved, with less use of inspiratory speech. Her maximum phonation time was nine seconds, and not commensurate with her complaints of severe shortness of breath. On speech spectrogram measures, her only abnormalities were increased frequency of aperiodic phonation, reduced intensity range, and aphonia on utterances of increasing numbers of syllables.

During vital capacity testing, F.C. had a 50 percent reduction in expiratory flow and gasped several times while breathing into the spirometer. Rib cage and abdominal movement signals were recorded with the Respitrace during quiet breathing. Irregular and oppositional movements occurred in the two compartments. This pattern normalized when verbal directions were provided for inspiration and expiration. Signals recorded during the controlled speech testing were also uncoordinated and oppositional during sentence production at regular and slow rates, and improved somewhat during sentence imitation at a slow rate when she was using expiratory speech (Figure 15-1).

Extensive pulmonary testing done in November, 1986, demonstrated that peak flow rate, maximum volume, and gas diffusion rates were normal. Only expiratory flow was reduced, suggesting expiratory airway obstruction. Her shortness of breath was likely due to uncoordinated rib cage and

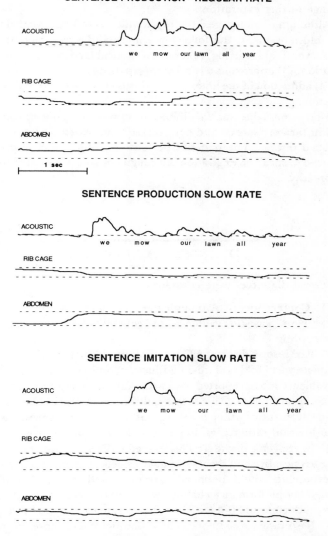

Figure 15-1. Acoustic amplitude, rib cage, and abdominal movement tracings during production of the same sentence in three speech conditions; at regular speech rate, at a self-paced slow rate, and during imitation of the examiner speaking at a slow rate. The dashed lines around each tracing are provided to emphasize the direction of the respiratory movement tracings. These movement signals are in arbitrary units. An upward excursion denotes ribcage or abdominal expansion, while a downward excursion denotes a decrease in cavity size.

abdominal movements and vocal fold adduction preventing sufficient air exchange during expiration.

Although nasolaryngeal fiberoptic videorecording revealed symmetric vocal fold movement, the following abnormalities were noted: (1) diffuse bilateral vocal fold scarring, (2) excessive vertical laryngeal movement during phonation, (3) approximately a 1 mm gap during adduction for phonation and, (4) adduction of the anterior two-thirds of the vocal folds during resting expiration.

Most remarkable was the difference between the patient's conversational use of inspiratory speech and her markedly improved performance during controlled testing. The patient's performance noticeably improved when instructed to speak on expiration, although her voice continued to be hoarse and breathy.

DIAGNOSTIC ALTERNATIVES

Several diagnoses were considered.

1. Contact ulcers: Although these are often associated with gastric reflux, there was no evidence of contact ulcers on the fiberoptic videorecording.

2. Parkinson's disease: F.C.'s expiratory adduction of the vocal folds, incomplete vocal fold closure on adduction, and respiratory flow problems are problems often reported in Parkinson's disease (Vincken, Gauthier, Dollfuss, et al., 1984). This seems unlikely, however, because she did not have involvement of other body regions, and her movement disorder was discoordination rather than movement slowness or rigidity.

3. Psychogenic disorder: This seemed unlikely because her psychosocial history was negative and she was an independent, confident, highly successful businesswoman who functioned extremely well despite her difficulties. Although her performance changed with speaking conditions, these changes were reproducible and did not alter when commented upon by the examiner.

4. Respiratory dyskinesia: These findings could represent respiratory dyskinesia with an associated laryngeal movement disorder because of her shortness of breath, uncoordinated rib cage and abdominal movements, and vocal fold adduction during expiration. All 10 cases of respiratory dyskinesia reported in the literature (Chiang, Pitts, & Rodriguez-Garcia, 1985) had tardive dyskinesia secondary to neuroleptic treatment for schizophrenia. Various forms of oral-lingual-buccal-facial or trunk and limb dyskinesia accompany this disorder, and only one case had an accompanying speech

disorder (Faheem, Brightwell, Burton, et al., 1982). This was described as "rhythmless or irregular volume with a loss of control of gross laryngeal adductory and abductory movement and fine vocal elasticity." Voice control and biofeedback were unsuccessful in that case, while reserpine, often used in phenothiazine-induced dyskinesia, was beneficial in the four cases where it was tried (Weiner, Goetz, Nausieda, & Klawans, 1978; Faheem et al., 1982). Symptoms characteristic of respiratory tardive dyskinesia are described as shortness of breath at rest, noisy breathing, an irregular breathing pattern, and gasps during inspiration.

5. Secondary to asthma: Another possibility was that her laryngeal and respiratory problems were secondary to her asthma. Electromyographic (EMG) recordings from the diaphragm, trunk, and neck muscles in asthmatics and controls have found increased activity in all muscles in asthmatics during breathing, even when both groups were using the same force. In addition, the pattern of muscle activation differed from normal. The asthmatics had a marked increase in activity in all their muscles simultaneous with inspiration onset and reduced muscle activity during expiration (Grønbæk & Skouby, 1960).

PHYSIOLOGICAL TESTING

We decided to examine F.C.'s respiratory and laryngeal physiology in more detail. She returned for laryngeal EMG. Bipolar concentric needle electrodes were inserted into the right and left thyroarytenoid muscles and the right and left cricothyroid muscles. Positions were validated with verifying gestures. The sum of the rib and abdominal movements from the Respitrace were recorded on Frequency Modulated (FM) tape, along with the speech signal.

The EMG signals were digitized at 2500 Hz and converted into microvolts using a linear regression equation based on a 2 volt calibration tone. The signals were full-wave rectified and smoothed with a 20 ms lag filter after measuring and subtracting impedence noise. To determine whether the laryngeal muscles were hyperactive, the minimum activation levels (during quiet respiration) and the maximum activation levels (during effort closure and swallow) were measured in microvolts. The beginning of the inspiratory and expiratory respiratory cycles were marked from visual inspection of the Respitrace signal. The respiratory signal was slower than normal, irregular, and had sustained thyroarytenoid activity during both inspiration and expiration. Cricothyroid activity increased just prior to inspiration (Figure 15-2).

RESPIRATION AT BASELINE

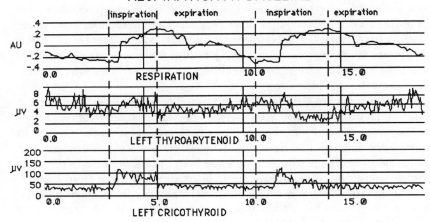

RESPIRATION

LEFT THYROARYTENOID

LEFT CRICOTHYROID

SENTENCE PRODUCTION AT BASELINE

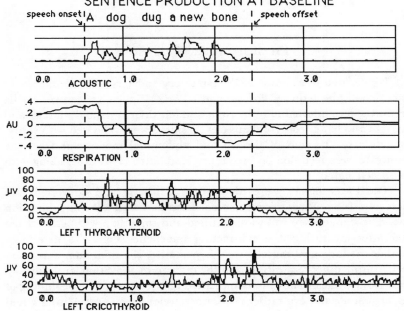

ACOUSTIC

RESPIRATION

LEFT THYROARYTENOID

LEFT CRICOTHYROID

when the EMG signal increased 200 percent above the minimum level was identified automatically, verified by visual inspection, and marked as the time of initiation of muscle activation prior to speech. Similarly, the time of muscle activation offset was marked when the muscle decreased to minimum levels, and was verified by visual inspection. The mean muscle activity between muscle activation onset and offset was computed. This mean was then divided by the maximum activation level measured during effort closure and swallow for that muscle to determine the percent of maximum. The mean percent of maximum activation for three repetitions of sustained phonation and three repetitions of the sentence "a dog dug a new bone," were compared with the normal control's values. The percent of maximum activation was significantly increased (p < .01) for all four muscles in comparison with the control using the Mann-Whitney U Test (Figure 15-4). Therefore, hyperactive activation patterns were found in the cricothyroid muscles during respiration and in both the thyroarytenoid and cricothyroid muscles during speech.

TREATMENT

These findings of muscle hyperactivity were indicative of a dystonia. Following a neurological consultation the patient was placed on anticholinergic therapy in March, 1987. During the first week on trihexyphenidyl hydrochloride (Artane), she reported fatigue and did not perceive a benefit. When the dosage was increased to 4 mg, she noticed a marked improvement in her breathing problems. She was speaking on expiration and no longer had a feeling of shortness of breath or episodes of aphonia. Although her voice quality continued to be hoarse and somewhat breathy, she no longer had difficulty with communication on the telephone.

She returned for reevaluation in September, 1987. The laryngeal EMG and respiratory movement study was repeated. Her respiratory pattern was now regular and at a more rapid normal rate. Thyroarytenoid and cricothyroid muscle activations were now synchronous and coincident with

Figure 15-2. Samples of physiological signals recorded at baseline. The sum Respitrace signal in arbitrary units (AU) shows the sum of rib cage and abdominal movement during quiet respiration. The simultaneous electromyographic signals for the left thyroarytenid and cricothyroid muscles are shown in microvolts following rectification and smoothing. The inspiration and expiration cycles are marked with hatched vertical lines, and the y-axis is in seconds. The same signals are shown during production of a sentence. The speech amplitude tracing has been full wave rectified and is in arbitrary units.

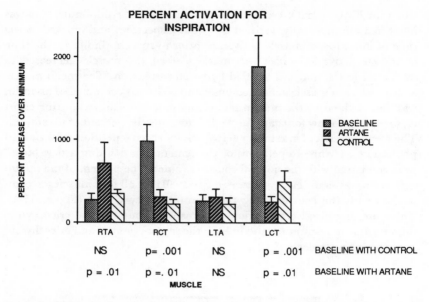

Figure 15-3. Mean percent increase in muscle activation for each muscle for the inspiratory cycles for F.C. at baseline testing and while on Artane and for the age- and sex-matched control. The bars show the mean value, while the lines show one standard deviation for the same data set. The probabilities resulting from Mann-Whitney U computations are shown for comparisons between F.C.'s baseline data and the normal control, and between F.C.'s baseline and Artane data.

TREATMENT

These findings of muscle hyperactivity were indicative of a dystonia. Following a neurological consultation the patient was placed on anticholinergic therapy in March, 1987. During the first week on trihexyphenidyl hydrochloride (Artane), she reported fatigue and did not perceive a benefit. When the dosage was increased to 4 mg, she noticed a marked improvement in her breathing problems. She was speaking on expiration and no longer had a feeling of shortness of breath or episodes of aphonia. Although her voice quality continued to be hoarse and somewhat breathy, she no longer had difficulty with communication on the telephone.

She returned for reevaluation in September, 1987. The laryngeal EMG and respiratory movement study was repeated. Her respiratory pattern was now regular and at a more rapid normal rate. Thyroarytenoid and cricothyroid muscle activations were now synchronous and coincident with inspiration (Figure 15-5). Measures of the percentage of increase in muscle activation with inspiration were significantly reduced ($p \leq .01$) in the

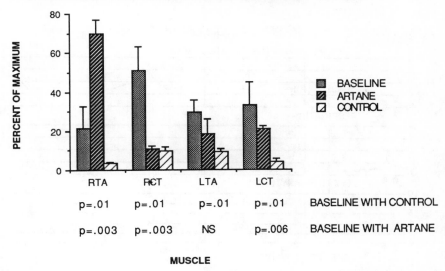

PERCENT OF MAXIMUM ACTIVATION DURING SPEECH

Figure 15-4. Mean percent of maximum muscle activation for each muscle for phonation and sentence production for F.C. at baseline testing and while on Artane and for the age- and sex-matched control. The bars show the mean value, while the lines show one standard deviation for the same data set. The probabilities resulting from Mann-Whitney U computations are shown for comparisons between F.C.'s baseline data and the normal control, and between F.C.'s baseline and Artane data.

cricothyroid muscles and increased in the right thyroarytenoid muscle when compared with measures made at baseline (Figure 15-3). Speech was now expiratory and accompanied activation in both the cricothyroid and thyroarytenoid muscles during phonation (Figure 15-5). The mean percent of maximum activation was measured in all four muscles during extended phonation; speech and was significantly decreased in the cricothyroid muscles and significantly increased in the right thyroarytenoid (Figure 15-4). This last comparison was the only significant change with Artane that was not in the direction of the values for the normal control.

EFFECTS OF IMPROVING RESPIRATORY CONTROL ON SPEECH PRODUCTION

To determine whether treatment of F.C.'s respiratory motor control disorder improved her speech production, objective comparisons were made between measures made from her pre- and post-treatment speech recordings. Her mean maximum phonation length increased from 9 to 12 seconds, and

RESPIRATION ON ARTANE

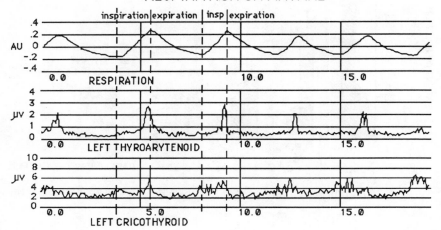

SENTENCE PRODUCTION ON ARTANE

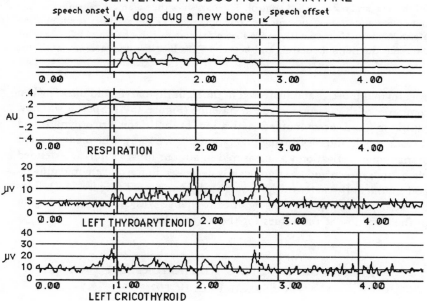

phonation on/off rates increased from 11 to 15 in 10 seconds. Mean jitter and shimmer measures were made from F.C.'s extended phonations using a dedicated hardware and software processing system previously described (Ludlow, Bassich, Connor, et al., 1986). Although mean jitter and shimmer measures were reduced from 1,280 μs to 968 μs, and from 15 percent to 10 percent respectively, these were still outside the normal range, indicating that some abnormality persisted.

At baseline, F.C. was aphonic on sentences of increasing length. We measured the duration of aperiodic phonation from sound spectrograms in sentences of increasing length. At baseline, the percent of her phonation that was aperiodic was increased as sentences increased in length (Figure 15-6). Following treatment the percent of aperiodic phonation was decreased overall and the percent aperiodicity did not increase with increasing sentence length.

Finally, to determine whether changes in speech performance associated with treatment of F.C.'s respiratory problem improved her speech and voice disorder, videotapes of reading (a highly structured speech task) and conversational speech, before and after treatment, were spliced without patient or condition identification. An experienced speech–language pathologist rated the two segments on the videotape blind to condition, using the 38 items contained in the rating scale of Darley, Aronson, and Brown (1968). F.C. had a rating of 2 or greater on 19 items at baseline. Most impaired were breathy voice (continuous) and voice stoppages, with a rating of 6, while bizarreness, pitch breaks, monopitch, harsh voice, strain-strangle, and inappropriate silences had ratings of 4 or 5. While on Artane, only five items were rated as impaired. Voice tremor increased from normal to a 3, while pitch breaks, breathy voice, voice stoppages, and bizarreness were all reduced to a 2 rating.

DISCUSSION

F.C.'s respiratory and EMG test results suggest she had dystonia. Her respiratory movements were dyskinetic and the heightened activations of her

---

Figure 15-5. Samples of physiological signals recorded on Artane. The sum Respitrace signal in arbitrary units (AU) shows the sum of rib cage and abdominal movement during quiet respiration. The simultaneous electromyographic signals for the left thyroarytenid and cricothyroid muscles are shown in microvolts following rectification and smoothing. The inspiration and expiration cycles are marked with hatched vertical lines and the y-axis is in seconds. The same signals are shown during production of a sentence. The speech amplitude tracing has been full-wave rectified and is in arbitrary units.

laryngeal muscles were similar to those seen in spasmodic dysphonia (Ludlow, Baker, Naunton, et al., 1987). Her laryngeal symptoms were not typical of spasmodic dysphonia, however, because no evidence of adductory spasms or overcontraction were seen on fiberoptic nasolaryngeal videorecording when F.C. was speaking on expiration. The improvement in her speech and voice functioning following improvement in her respiratory movement control and reduction in laryngeal muscle activation suggests that the laryngeal and respiratory dystonia were the basis for her speech symptoms. Her response to Artane was very marked and not commensurate with our experience in patients with spasmodic dysphonia.

We are not able to rule out the possibility that F.C.'s movement disorder could be psychogenic, because we did not use a sham treatment trial such as administration of a placebo form of Artane. However, several factors suggest that her disorder was not psychogenic. First, she did not have an initial response to treatment and received a benefit only when the dosage was increased. Second, over one year since treatment was initiated, her symptoms have not returned and continue to be controlled at the same dosage level. She has not received any other forms of treatment during this time. Often in a psychogenic disorder, treatment benefits without insight by the patient are short-lived.

No information is available on the basis for FC's movement disorder.

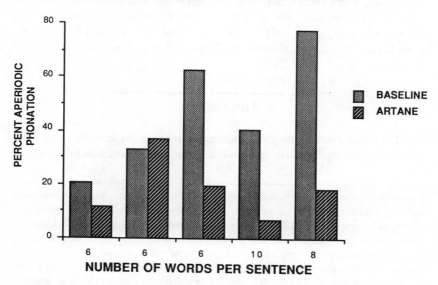

Figure 15-6. The percent of phonation that was aperiodic is plotted for each of five sentences produced by F.C. at baseline testing and when on 4 mg of Artane.

Consideration should be given to the frequency of respiratory movements used by patients with severe asthma in response to their increased airway resistance. In addition, the use of inhalants requires the use of a particular motor gesture involving forced expiration, followed by spraying during inspiration and effort closure. Therefore, F.C. was using excessive respiratory posturing that could constitute a motor overuse syndrome, such as occurs in writer's or musician's cramp.

Based on our findings with F.C., we would recommend attention to respiratory and laryngeal coordination during diagnostic assessment of a patient who demonstrates speech on inspiration and complains of shortness of breath.

ACKNOWLEDGMENTS

The authors wish to thank Dr. Sheila Stager for perceptual assessment of the videotaped samples and editorial comments, and Celia Bassich for conducting the acoustic analyses of jitter and shimmer.

REFERENCES

Chiang, E., Pitts, W.M., & Rodriguez-Garcia, M. (1985). Respiratory dyskinesia: Review and case reports. *Journal of Clinical Psychiatry, 46*, 232-234.

Darley, F., Aronson, A., & Brown, J. (1968). Differential diagnosis patterns of dysarthria. *Journal of Speech and Hearing Research, 12*, 246-269.

Faheem, A.D., Brightwell, D.R., Burton, G.C., & Struss, A. (1982). Respiratory dyskinesia and dysarthria from prolonged neuroleptic use: Tardive dyskinesia? *American Journal of Psychiatry, 139*(4), 517-518.

Grønbæk, P. & Skouby, A.P. (1960). The activity pattern of the diaphragm and some muscles of the neck and trunk in chronic asthmatics and normal controls: A comparative electromyographic study. *Acta Medicus Scandinavia, 168*(5-6), 413-425.

Ludlow, C.L., Baker, M., Naunton, R.F., & Hallett, M. (1987). Intrinsic laryngeal muscle activation in spasmodic dysphonia. In R. Benecke, B. Conrad & C.D. Marsden (Eds.), *Motor disturbances I*. Orlando, FL: Academic Press.

Ludlow, C.L., Bassich, C.J., Connor, N.P., Coulter, D.A., & Lee, Y.J. (1986). The validity of using phonatory jitter and shimmer to detect laryngeal pathology. In T. Baer, C. Sasaski, & K. Harris (Eds.), *Laryngeal function in phonation and respiration*. San Diego: College-Hill Press.

Vincken, W.G., Gauthier, S.G., Dollfuss, R.E., Hanson, R.E., Darauay, C.M., & Cosio, M.G. (1984). Involvement of upper-airway muscles in extrapyramidal disorders: A cause of airflow limitation. *New England Journal of Medicine, 311*(7), 438-441.

Weiner, W.J., Goetz, C.G., Nausieda, P.A., & Klawans, H.L. (1978). Respiratory dyskinesias: Extrapyramidal dysfunction and dyspnea. *Annals of Internal Medicine, 88*, 327-331.

CHAPTER 16

KATHRYN M. YORKSTON

FACIAL ANASTAMOSIS IN A DYSARTHRIC SPEAKER

*D*ifferential diagnosis was not an issue in the case that will be described in this chapter, but the editors have asked that it be included because it presents a clinical quandary. In this case, the diagnosis was clearly a brainstem cerebrovascular accident (CVA) with involvement of seventh cranial nerve, which resulted in paralysis of the right side of the face. The medical team had to predict the consequences of a surgical procedure that would, on one hand, increase the level of impairment by partially altering tongue innervation and, on the other hand, decrease the cosmetic and speech problems associated with unilateral facial paralysis. The specific question faced by the medical team was, Should a seventh to twelfth cranial nerve anastomosis be performed in a dysarthric woman?

An anastomosis is the surgical connection of a portion of one cranial nerve, in this case the twelfth, or hypoglossal, to the seventh, or facial, nerve. Such a procedure is schematically illustrated in Figure 16-1. Note that presurgically there is lack of innervation to the right side of the face because of damage to nerve supplying that area. Postsurgically, this innervation is reestablished through the twelfth cranial nerve.

Moderately successful rehabilitation of facial muscle paralysis of a peripheral nature has been reported for a number of years (Booker, Rubow, & Coleman, 1969; and Daniel & Guitar, 1978). For example, Hammerschlag, Brudny, Cusumano, and Cohen (1987) studied the effects of hypoglossal-facial nerve anastomosis, with and without postoperative EMG rehabilitation, on a group of 16 people. Results indicated a trend toward better outcomes in the group with EMG feedback training. The majority of patients

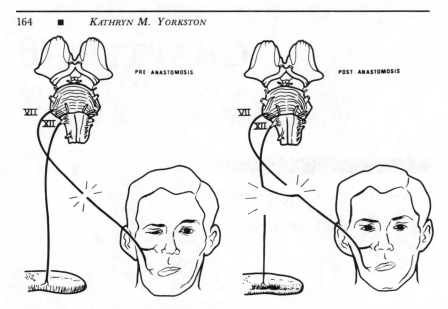

Figure 16-1. A schematic representation of a seventh to twelfth cranial nerve anastomosis. From B. Daniel and B. Guitar (1978). EMG feedback and recovery of facial and speech gestures following neural anastomosis. *Journal of Speech and Hearing Disorders, 43,* 705–709. Reprinted with permission.

who undergo hypoglossal-facial nerve anastomosis are not experiencing involvement of the tongue prior to surgery. None of the subjects reviewed in previous research reports was said to be dysarthric presurgically. Despite apparently normal lingual function presurgically, some minor consequences for tongue movement as it relates to speech have been noted. Daniel and Guitar described the postsurgical consequences for the case they reported, a person who was free of lingual involvement prior to surgery.

> Speech was perceptually normal except for a slight distortion when he rapidly uttered triple blends. . . . Interestingly, the loss of half of the tongue's innervation produced more of a cosmetic difference during speech than an auditory-perceptual one. (p. 11)

Despite the reports of good compensation by individuals with no lingual involvement prior to surgery, the presence of pre-existing dysarthria complicates the decision whether or not to recommend surgery. The management team along with the patient must weigh the relative benefits of reinnervation to the face and possible consequences for removing a portion of the innervation to the tongue.

DESCRIPTION OF THE CASE

M.C. was a 32-year-old college graduate and 8 months pregnant when she experienced a severe brainstem CVA. Initial hospitalization and rehabilitation was completed at another facility, but medical records and patient reports indicated that initially she was only able to move her eyes. This was followed by a gradual recovery of function. She was first evaluated in the Department of Rehabilitation Medicine, University of Washington, at 12 months post-onset in preparation for her relocation to the Seattle area. At this time, speech production was characterized by adequate respiratory support with a sustained phonation time of over 10 seconds. M.C. was velopharyngeally competent in that she was able to generate adequate intraoral air pressure during the production of pressure consonants, and her speech was not excessive hypernasal. Oral articulatory movements were mildly to moderately imprecise. Sentence intelligibility at that time was measured to be 80 percent at a speaking rate of just over 80 words per minute (wpm) (Yorkston, Beukelman, & Traynor, 1984). Thus M.C. had progressed, in the first year post-onset, from no functional speech to a point at which she was considered a functional but slow speaker.

At 19 months post-onset, she relocated to Seattle and was reevaluated. During the intervening period, she had continued to receive regular speech treatment, with a focus on improving articulatory precision. Results of the evaluation at 19 months post-onset indicated that her intelligibility had improved to 92 percent intelligible at the same speaking rate. At the time of her relocation to Seattle, she was evaluated in the Department of Otolaryngology for possible surgery in an effort to reduce her residual right facial paralysis.

CONSIDERATIONS WHEN EVALUATING POTENTIAL FOR SURGERY

POSITIVE INDICATORS

A number of factors suggested that surgery was warranted. First, the cosmetic aspects of facial paralysis were unacceptable for this young mother. She also faced the possibility of future decrease of labial function with continued muscular atrophy. Thus, with increasing atrophy, bilabial function related to speech might worsen and affect overall speech performance. Finally, M.C. was an intelligent woman who had already demonstrated good compensatory skills related to speech production. She was well motivated to continue work on speech.

Cautions

Cautions were necessary regarding the recommendations to undergo the surgery related to speech. What would be the consequences of decreasing innervation to the tongue in a woman who, with considerable effort, had just reached the point at which she felt she could be easily understood by a listener who was unfamiliar with her? Although she was now 90 percent intelligible, she was still speaking at approximately one-half of a normal rate.

Because the team was very concerned about the decrease in tongue innervation for this patient who already needed to compensate for tongue involvement, an effort was made to mimic the surgery in a temporary fashion by means of a temporary nerve block to the twelfth cranial nerve. Unfortunately, the block did not successfully deaden the nerve, so the experiment was nonconclusive. Nonetheless, the patient and her husband decided to proceed with the surgery.

Results of the Surgery

Measures of Speech Performance

Figure 16-2 illustrates sentence intelligibility over time with surgical anastomosis occurring approximately 20 months post-onset. Note that the first reassessment two months after surgery indicated a reduction in intelligibility from 92 to 72 percent. This reduction in intelligibility was accompanied by a slight reduction in speaking rate, from 85 to 78 wpm. With weekly speech treatment sessions emphasizing maintenance of an appropriate speaking rate and precise production of lingual sounds, speech intelligibility returned to presurgical level, and perhaps a bit higher.

Results of an evaluation of consonant production before and after surgery are illustrated in Figure 16-3. An examination of the figure suggests that the pattern of decrease after surgery followed by improvement to presurgical levels is similar to the pattern seen in speech intelligibility measures. Consonant production was characterized by a predictable pattern of change, with lingual consonants being the most severely affected immediately after surgery. Categories most affected were lingual-velar stops, fricatives, and affricates. Difficulty managing saliva initially made production of the fricative and affricates difficult. The course of recovery of

ASSESSMENT OF INTELLIGIBILITY OF DYSARTHRIC SPEECH
RATE/INTELLIGIBILITY GRAPH

Speaker: **M.C.**   #: **UH**   Date of Onset: **3/85**

Type of Dysarthria: **FLACCID**   Etiology: **BRAINSTEM CVD**

Key		
W-MC	Multiple Choice Style Word Intelligibility	I Intelligible Words Per Minute
W-T	Single Word Transcription Intelligibility	U Unintelligible Words Per Minute
S	Sentence Intelligibility	—
R	Speaking Rate	—

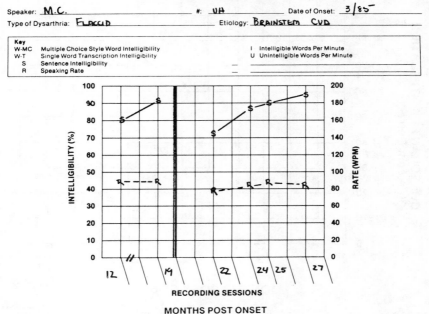

RECORDING SESSIONS

MONTHS POST ONSET

Figure 16-2. Sentence intelligibility and speaking rates for M.C. from 12 through 27 months post-onset (Yorkston, Beukelman, & Traynor, 1984).

phoneme production ability paralleled the return of speech intelligibility to presurgical levels, with the last phonemes to reappear being the lingual-velar stops.

SUBJECTIVE REPORTS

M.C. felt her level of articulatory precision decreased immediately following surgery. At least in the first months after surgery, she needed to monitor her speech more closely than prior to the surgery. Speech was made more difficult to understand because of her increased difficulty managing her saliva. The team was somewhat surprised to note that her chief complaint following the surgery was not the effects on speech but on swallowing. In the initial months following the surgery, she reported that the oral phase swallowing was much more laborious; that her eating time had at least doubled as compared to before the surgery; and, that a conscious effort was needed to manage saliva.

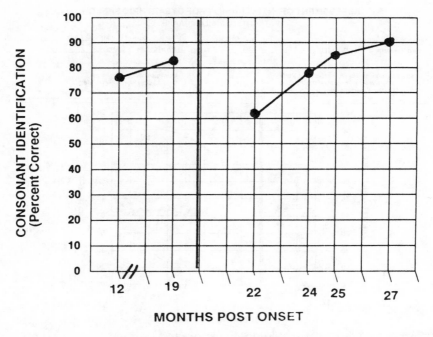

Figure 16-3. Consonant identification scores from the Phoneme Identification Task (Yorkston, Beukelman, & Traynor, in press) for M.C. from 12 through 27 months post-onset.

DISCUSSION

M.C. has now been followed for approximately one year after her surgery. Most indicators point to a positive outcome. The surgery was successful in improving facial symmetry and muscle tone. Results of EMG studies show some reinnervation of facial muscles. Some trace movement on the right side can be noted with smiling and simultaneous tongue elevation. Further, anticipated losses in articulatory precision were temporary. Speech has returned to presurgery levels, although it has not progressed beyond those levels. The swallowing and saliva management difficulties have been resolved.

In reviewing the case of M.C., it is clear that a number of factors may have contributed to the successful outcome. These factors may be useful in suggesting candidacy guidelines for such intervention with similar cases. First, M.C. was a functional verbal communicator prior to surgery. Although obviously dysarthric, her speech intelligibility was over 90 percent. The type of surgical intervention described here should be approached with extreme caution with those who are more severely involved than M.C. There was an obvious increase in the level of impairment following surgery. This increased impairment was also associated with a temporary increase in the level of disability and a reduction in speech intelligibility. It is an open question whether or not people with impairments more severe than that of M.C. could compensate as well as she. Second, M.C. was cognitively intact and well-motivated. These characteristics would also appear to be mandatory for candidates for this procedure, because compensatory adjustments are required in the face of increasing lingual involvement.

Finally, close association between changes in speech impairment and increasing difficulty in swallowing and saliva management should be expected. The co-occurrence of speech and swallowing difficulties in patients with lingual involvement has been reported in the literature (Hillel & Miller, in press; and Logemann, 1983). Altered innervation to the tongue increases difficulty in the oral phase of swallowing. M.C. reported that bolus management was more difficult and the time required for eating increased greatly. Increased lingual involvement also resulted in more difficulty with saliva management. M.C. indicated that in the months immediately following the surgery she continually needed to make a conscious effort to swallow saliva. Thus presurgical counseling should not only prepare the potential candidate for changes in speech, but also changes in swallowing abilities.

ACKNOWLEDGMENTS

This article was supported in part by Grant # G008200020 from the National Institute of Disability and Rehabilitation Research, Department of Education, Washington, D.C.

REFERENCES

Booker, H.E., Rubow, R.T., & Coleman, P.J. (1969). Simplified feedback in neuromuscular retraining: An automatic approach using electromyographic signals. *Archives of Physical Medicine and Rehabilitation, 50,* 621-625.

Daniel, B., & Guitar, B. (1978). EMG feedback and recovery of facial and speech gestures following neural anastomosis. *Journal of Speech and Hearing Disorders, 43,* 9-20.

Hammerschlag, P.E., Brudny, J., Cusumano, R., & Cohen, N.L. (1987). Hypoglossal-facial nerve anastomosis and electromyographic feedback rehabilitation. *Laryngoscope, 97,* 705-709.

Hillel, A.D., & Miller, R.M. (in press). Bulbar amyotrophic lateral sclerosis: Patterns of progression and clinical management. *Head and Neck Surgery.*

Logemann, J. (1983). *Evaluation and treatment of swallowing disorders.* San Diego: College-Hill Press.

Yorkston, K.M., Beukelman, D.R., & Bell, K.R. (1988). *Clinical management of dysarthric speakers.* San Diego: College-Hill Press.

Yorkston, K.M., Beukelman, D.R., & Traynor, C.D. (1984). *Computerized assessment of intelligibility of dysarthric speech.* Austin, TX: ProEd.

Yorkston, K.M., Beukelman, D.R., & Traynor, C.D. (in press). Articulatory adequacy in dysarthric speakers: A comparison of judging formats. *Journal of Communication Disorders.*

SECTION VII

DIAGNOSING DEMENTIA IN PATIENTS WITH EARLY ONSET OF SPEECH-LANGUAGE PROBLEMS

CHAPTER 17

KATHRYN A. BAYLES
CHERYL K. TOMOEDA

███████████████████

EVIDENCE OF A
DEMENTING DISEASE IN
AN APHASIC STROKE
PATIENT?

A 68-year-old man referred himself to the Veteran's Administration Medical Center because of recurrent headaches in the occipital region. The headaches occurred five to eight times daily and were associated with nausea and vomiting. Two years earlier this man, who will be referred to as Mr. K., participated in a research project conducted by us. Because of a history of cerebrovascular accident (CVA), he served as a subject in a stroke group whose performance on a variety of neuropsychological tasks was compared to performances of people with mild and moderate Alzheimer's disease (AD) and normal elders. When Mr. K. developed recurrent headaches, information about his neuropsychological history became of interest, and our research team was contacted to provide Mr. K.'s early performance data. The symptomatology reported by Mr. K., and the changes in his neuropsychological status, led his physicians to consider the following diagnoses: vascular dementia, Alzheimer's disease, subcortical dementia, a mass lesion, or depression.

─────────────────────

BRIEF HISTORY OF CASE

Mr. K., a retired carpenter, was right-handed, married, and spoke English as his first language. In 1980, he suffered a CVA that resulted in the development of a hematoma which was evacuated via craniotomy. The CT scan taken prior to the craniotomy revealed,

> in the supratentorial compartment, a 3 × 4.8 cm area of increased density . . . in the left temporal lobe. This is assumed to be a hematoma. This is producing a 6 mm shift of midline structures from left to right. The left lateral ventricle is effaced. A slight amount of edema surrounds the area of the hematoma.

Six months after the craniotomy, Mr. K. was evaluated by a neuro-psychologist who reported cognitive deficits and emotional disturbance. Specifically, Mr. K. was described as having "weak short-term verbal recall," "poor delayed recall for verbal information," but "excellent tactile and spatial memory." Further, he was reported as having "weak abstract conceptualiza-tion skills" and "problem-solving deficits." Finally, the neuropsychologist reported evidence of "depression, anxiety, and confusion."

Five and a half years after the neuropsychological evaluation, Mr. K. was recruited for participation in a comparative study of the performance of stroke and AD patients on a variety of neuropsychological tasks. As part of his participation, Mr. K. was given the Western Aphasia Battery (WAB) (Kertesz, 1982) to determine the presence and type of aphasia. He obtained an aphasia quotient of 89.2, indicative of mild aphasia, and the pattern of performance typified anomic aphasia. In addition, Mr. K. was given a speech discrimination test which he completed with 100 percent accuracy, indicating hearing sufficiently good for reliably completing the tasks in the research protocol.

The neuropsychological tasks administered as part of the research study included tests of mental status, memory, oral description, reading com-prehension, linguistic disambiguation, pantomime expression, generative naming, and drawing. Mr. K.'s test performance scores are shown in Table 17-1, where they may be compared to the mean performance scores of mild and moderate AD patients, other aphasic stroke patients, and normal elders.

Comparison of Mr. K.'s Performance to that of AD Patients

With two exceptions Mr. K. did not perform as the mild or moderate AD patients on the tasks used in the research project; he performed better. The two scores that were close to the means of mild AD patients were observed on the story-retelling task in the immediate condition and the FAS Word Fluency Measure (Borkowski, Benton, & Spreen, 1967), two measures particularly sensitive to mild dementia (Bayles & Kaszniak, 1987). In Alzheimer's dementia, however, a poor performance on these tasks is associated with a correspondingly poor performance on the mental status task. Such was not the case with Mr. K., whose mental status score was nearly normal. The poorer performance of Mr. K. on the story-retelling and Word Fluency tasks, in the absence of mental status deficits, may be explained instead by the mild aphasia demonstrated in his WAB performance.

COMPARISON OF MR. K.'S PERFORMANCE TO THAT OF APHASIC STROKE PATIENTS

When compared with aphasic stroke patients, Mr. K. was superior in performance on oral description, reading comprehension, sentence disambiguation, the FAS Word Fluency Measure, and story-retelling in the delayed condition. The four tasks on which he was inferior in performance to other aphasic stroke patients were story-retelling in the immediate condition, delayed spatial recognition memory, delayed verbal recognition memory, and drawing. The first three of these tasks depend in large part on episodic memory function; that is, the ability to recall information in context. A synonym for episodic memory is contextual memory. In the story-retelling—immediate condition task, the individual must remember the event of the story and retell it; in the delayed spatial recognition memory task, the individual must remember the episodic exposure of a visuospatial context; and in the delayed verbal recognition memory task, the individual must remember the episodic exposure of a group of words.

SECOND NEUROPSYCHOLOGICAL HISTORY

Because of the advent of new neurological symptoms eight years after Mr. K.'s CVA, his physicians became interested in his neuropsychological history. Thus, in addition to a neurological evaluation, a second neuropsychological evaluation was scheduled, and a request was made of us to readminister the research protocol given two years earlier.

RESULTS OF SECOND NEUROLOGICAL EVALUATION

A CT scan was performed and showed that in addition to the old infarct and craniotomy, "some mild degenerative changes [were present] in the deep cerebral white matter bilaterally, particularly in the parietal regions. With no evidence of supratentorial mass." Mr. K. had a residual mild right-sided hemiparesis, but did not suffer from diplopia, dysarthria, fever, chills, loss of consciousness, or seizures. He was noted to have a history of cervical spine disease beginning four years after the documented CVA. Results of EEG, when awake and during sleep, indicated "some slowing in the left temporal-parietal region."

TABLE 17-1.
Raw scores and Z-scores of Mr. K. across two test sessions.

Test Given (Raw Scores)	Healthy Elderly: Mean; SD (Z-Score Conversion)	Mild AD: Mean; SD (Z-Score Conversion)	Moderate AD: Mean; SD (Z-Score Conversion)	Nonfluent Aphasia: Mean; SD (Z-Score Conversion)	Fluent Aphasia: Mean; SD (Z-Score Conversion)
Mental Status	12.87; 0.34	6.81; 2.99	2.41; 2.68	9.18; 3.79	10.83; 3.20
T-1 = 12	-2.56	1.74	3.58	0.74	0.37
T-2 = 10	-8.44	1.07	2.83	0.22	-0.26
Story-retelling—Immediate	19.81; 2.99	9.33; 5.09	3.03; 3.89	11.67; 3.56	15.29; 3.72
T-1 = 10	-3.28	0.13	1.79	-0.47	-1.42
T-2 = 18	-0.61	1.70	3.85	1.78	0.73
Delayed Spatial Recognition Memory	10.24; 2.67	3.33; 1.98	2.05; 2.39	7.88; 3.98	8.80; 2.71
T-1 = 8	-0.84	2.36	2.49	0.03	-0.30
T-2 = 8	-0.84	2.36	2.49	0.03	-0.30
Delayed Verbal Recognition Memory	11.41; 2.61	3.00; 2.37	1.58; 1.87	7.25; 5.08	8.88; 3.62
T-1 = 6	-2.10	1.27	2.36	-0.25	-0.80
T-2 = 8	-1.33	2.11	3.43	0.15	-0.24

	C1	C2	C3	C4	C5
Oral Object Description					
T1 = 34	42.57; 18.68	15.48; 9.69	5.70; 6.99	8.40; 3.36	20.45; 10.14
T2 = NA	-0.46	1.91	4.05	7.62	1.34
Total Reading Comprehension					
T1 = 16	17.21; 1.29	11.19; 2.80	5.47; 4.05	10.94; 4.04	13.76; 3.33
	-0.94	1.72	2.60	1.25	0.67
T2 = 10	-5.59	-0.42	1.12	-0.23	-1.13
Total Sentence Disambiguation					
T1 = 6	7.67; 1.95	2.29; 2.22	0.83; 1.40	2.86; 2.93	5.09; 2.37
T2 = NA	-0.86	1.67	3.69	1.07	0.38
Pantomime Expression					
T1 = 35	39.03; 9.78	17.14; 9.06	10.81; 10.86	23.69; 13.71	32.84; 11.38
	-0.41	1.97	2.23	0.82	0.19
T2 = 28	-1.13	1.20	1.58	0.31	-0.43
Drawing					
T1 = 13	18.74; 3.63	9.90; 5.54	3.73; 4.38	12.56; 5.59	15.28; 3.98
	-1.58	0.56	2.12	0.08	-0.57
T2 = 15	-1.03	0.92	2.57	0.44	-0.07
FAS Word Fluency Measure					
T1 = 17	39.48; 12.55	15.90; 12.03	4.89; 5.93	3.60; 4.30	10.87; 9.13
	-1.79	0.09	2.04	3.12	0.67
T2 = 17	-1.79	0.09	2.04	3.12	0.67
Story-retelling—Delayed					
T1 = 17	18.90; 3.31	0.19; 0.87	0.30; 1.39	9.17; 5.23	12.57; 6.17
	-0.57	19.32	12.01	1.50	0.72
T2 = 16	-0.88	18.17	11.29	1.31	0.56

Key: AD = Alzheimer's disease; SD = standard deviation; T-1 = first test; T-2 = second test; NA = not administered.

177

RESULTS OF SECOND NEUROPSYCHOLOGICAL EVALUATION

At the time of retesting, Mr. K. was found to be oriented to time and place. His remote memory was described as poor, as were his calculation and abstract reasoning skills. He was unable to follow a two-step command. His WAIS-R (Wechsler, 1981) Performance IQ was 101, Verbal IQ was 81, and Full-Scale IQ was 87. These scores were said to represent a mild decline since Mr. K.'s previous neuropsychological evaluation seven and one-half years earlier. A moderate decline in mental flexibility, problem solving, visuospatial tracking, and sequential reasoning was noted. As was the case in his previous neuropsychological evaluation, the patient appeared depressed.

RESULTS OF THE SECOND ADMINISTRATION OF THE RESEARCH PROTOCOL

Shortly after the second neuropsychological test, some of the tasks used in the research study were readministered. The full protocol was not given because Mr. K. complained of a headache and declined to continue the evaluation midway in the session. The performance scores at the second test time are shown in Table 17-1.

Mr. K.'s score on the mental status task was now lower, similar to that of aphasic patients, but higher than that of mild and moderate AD patients. A review of his answers showed that orientation to time and place was good, but simple questions of general knowledge were missed. Also lower were his scores on reading comprehension, pantomime expression, and story-retelling—delayed. Yet Mr. K.'s performance did not deteriorate on all tasks. He improved in performance on story-retelling in the immediate condition, in delayed verbal recognition memory, and in drawing. Unchanged were his performances on the delayed spatial recognition memory task and the FAS Word Fluency Measure.

A striking feature of Mr. K.'s performance was its variability. He did not exhibit an across-the-board decline on all tasks, and indeed improved on some of the tasks that were most impaired at the time of the first administration of the research protocol. Further, some inconsistencies in his performance were apparent. For example, Mr. K.'s poorer performance on the reading comprehension task would suggest linguistic comprehension deficits, yet his performance on the story-retelling task in the immediate condition, another type of linguistic comprehension task, improved. Finally, Mr. K. was reported to be very slow in responding by both the examiner and his wife.

DISCUSSION

The variability of Mr. K.'s performance does not dismiss the existence of cognitive deficits and deterioration in mental status. In fact, the change in mental status, in conjunction with his new neurological symptoms, raise the possibility of a dementing disease, particularly in the absence of a second CVA or mass lesion. Dementia is a syndrome associated with many diseases and conditions and is definable as the chronic progressive deterioration of intellect, personality, memory, and communicative function secondary to central nervous system degenerative processes. The identification of a dementing disease in this case is a complex endeavor, because Mr. K.'s symptoms do not neatly fit descriptions of the common cortical and subcortical dementing diseases.

The most common dementing disease is Alzheimer's disease, which is characterized in the early stages by prominent semantic and episodic memory deficits (Bayles & Kaszniak, 1987). Such deficits are observable in tasks requiring the encoding of verbal material and its delayed recall. Although Mr. K. had encoding difficulties at the time of his participation in the research project, as demonstrated by a depressed score on story-retelling in the immediate condition, he did not have them two years later. Improvement in encoding ability is atypical of the AD patient, who suffers progressive deterioration of semantic memory. Further, Mr. K. failed to demonstrate deterioration in episodic memory function as measured by performance on the story-retelling task in the delayed condition. The scores for delayed recall at both test times vary by a single point.

Other dementing diseases that should be considered, given the constellation of symptoms of Mr. K., are progressive perisylvian disease (Kirshner, Webb, Kelly, & Wells, 1984; Mesulam, 1982; Wechsler, 1977) Pick's disease, Parkinson's disease, and early Binswanger's disease.

Mesulam (1982) reported six patients with progressive perisylvian atrophy in whom prominent aphasia, in the absence of stroke, was the presenting symptom. Two of these individuals ultimately became fully demented. Kirshner, Webb, Kelly, & Wells (1984) reported six dementia patients in whom language disturbance was an isolated initial symptom or prominent part of a more general cognitive deterioration in the absence of transient ischemic attack or stroke. The fact that Mr. K. had a stroke and developed mild aphasia does not preclude the possibility of the development of this condition. However, two important pieces of diagnostic evidence are lacking; worsening aphasia and no mention of perisylvian atrophy or ventricular dilation in the interpretation of the second CT scan.

Another uncommon dementing disease to be considered as the cause of the symptomatology of Mr. K. is Pick's disease. In this disease, Pick bodies, dense intracellular structures, occur primarily in the cortical cells in the temporal and frontal lobes. Less commonly, neuron loss and astrocytic gliosis are reported to occur to a variable extent in the basal ganglia, thalamus, and subthalamic nucleus (Cummings & Duchen, 1981). Pathology in these brain regions produce personality and emotional changes, and the behavior of affected individuals is often bizarre. Further, deterioration in mental status is observed, and secondary memory may not be as prominently impaired as other cognitive skills (Cummings & Benson, 1983). Mr. K. had emotional and mental status changes, and secondary memory was relatively preserved (as evaluated in the delayed retelling of a story). However, Mr. K. had not been reported to exhibit bizarre behavior, and he lacked certain of the other characteristics of Pick's disease, such as presence of repetitive speech, echolalia, and Kluver-Bucy syndrome (emotional blunting, hyperorality, hypersexuality, compulsion to explore surroundings, and sensory agnosia).

Parkinson's disease is associated with subcortical pathology in the basal ganglia, specifically the pars compacta of the substantia nigra, and loss of the neurotransmitter dopamine. As a result of structural and chemical changes in subcortical areas, affected individuals have difficulty initiating and stopping movement, as well as rigidity, rest tremor, bradykinesia, and intellectual deficits. Further, the chemical imbalances in the brains of affected individuals are associated with depression, often a presenting symptom.

Parkinson's disease in the early stages can be difficult to diagnose, and particularly in a person with a history of CVA, mild aphasia, and residual hemiparesis. The features of Mr. K.'s condition suggestive of Parkinson's disease were slowness, depression, variability in performance, and circumscribed cognitive deficits in the absence of a full dementia. On the other hand, Mr. K. did not exhibit certain of the other characteristic features of Parkinsonism; rigidity, slow shuffling gait, or a mask-like face. The motor symptoms of Parkinson's disease usually are seen unilaterally, a fact that may be obscured in the case of Mr. K. because of a right-sided residual hemiparesis. The large majority of Parkinson's patients suffer intellectual deficits that are particularly apparent on tasks requiring effortful processing, visuospatial function, and the tracking of sequentially presented information. Mr. K. appeared to have difficulty on these types of tasks. Because not all the symptomatology associated with Parkinson's disease is observable in the early stages, the possibility that Mr. K. had early Parkinson's disease cannot be ruled out.

Of the conditions considered thus far, Binswanger's disease (periventricular leukoencephalopathy) may be the most likely. Binswanger's disease is being recognized with increasing frequency by means of proton magnetic resonance imaging (MRI) (Roman, 1987), a procedure Mr. K. had not been given. When the disease is present, associated white-matter changes appear in MRI as an intense halo of periventricular hyperintensity. Patients with the disease typically have a history of hypertension, diabetes, cardiovascular disease, and repeated strokes. Changes in mood and behavior are prominent (Babikian & Ropper, 1987), frontal lobe signs commonly occur, and intellectual deficits are demonstrable. Mutism, bradykinesia, rigidity, and dysarthria can also be present.

As has been previously noted, Mr. K. had experienced changes in mood, intellectual function, and was slow in responding (bradykinesia), but he did not have rigidity or dysarthria. He did, however, have a history of hypertension and cardiovascular disease, though not diabetes. Finally, he had observable subcortical white matter changes on CT.

A possible cause of Mr. K.'s dementia-like symptomatology that has not been discussed is depression, and we would be remiss if it were not mentioned. Depressed elderly people have been reported to have memory impairment, slowness of response, disorientation, impaired attention, poor word list generation, and motor slowing (Cummings & Benson, 1983). All of these behaviors were present in Mr. K.

CONCLUSION

At the time of the writing of this report, Mr. K. lacks a firm diagnosis. An MRI scan has not been performed, although it has been recommended. Of the possible causes considered in this case, early Parkinson's disease or Binswanger's disease seem more likely than Alzheimer's disease, Pick's disease, and progressive periventricular atrophy. The process of considering the possible causes of Mr. K.'s neurological and neuropsychological symptoms demonstrates the complexity of identifying the existence of a dementing disease in an aging person with mild aphasia, chronic motor dysfunction, and depression. An MRI scan, and treatment for possible depression, might lead to a more certain diagnosis.

ACKNOWLEDGMENTS

This work was partially supported by grants from the Andrus Foundation and the National Institute of Mental Health.

REFERENCES

Babikian, V., & Ropper, A.H. (1987). Binswanger's disease: A review. *Stroke, 18*, 2–12.

Bayles, K.A., & Kaszniak, A.W. (1987). *Communication and cognition in normal aging and dementia.* San Diego: College-Hill Press.

Borkowski, J.G., Benton, A.L., & Spreen, O. (1967). Word fluency and brain damage. *Neuropsychologia, 5*, 135–140.

Cummings, J.L., & Benson, D.F. (1983). *Dementia: A clinical approach.* Boston: Buttersworth.

Cummings, J.L., & Duchen, L.W. (1981). The Kluver-Bucy syndrome in Pick disease. *Neurology, 31,* 1415–1422.

Kertesz, A. (1982). *Western aphasia battery.* New York: Grune & Stratton.

Kirshner, H.S., Webb, W.G., Kelly, M.P., & Wells, C.E. (1984). Language disturbance: An initial symptom of cortical degeneration and dementia. *Archives of Neurology, 41,* 491–496.

Mesulam, M-M. (1982). Slowly progressive aphasia without generalized dementia. *Annals of Neurology, 11,* 592–598.

Roman, G.C. (1987). Senile dementia of the Binswanger type. *AMA, 258,* 1782–1788.

Wechsler, A.F. (1977). Presenile dementia presenting as aphasia. *Journal of Neurology, Neurosurgery, and Psychiatry, 40,* 303–305.

Wechsler, D. (1981). *Wechsler Adult Intelligence Scale-Revised Manual.* New York: The Psychological Corporation.

CHAPTER 18

JENNIFER HORNER
JOHN E. RISKI

EARLY DEMENTIA OF UNKNOWN TYPE: MIXED CORTICAL-SUBCORTICAL DEMENTIA?

*I*n the Spring of 1986, the Center for Speech and Hearing Disorders at Duke University Medical Center received a consultation request from the Muscular Dystrophy Clinic regarding a 69-year-old female patient who was undergoing evaluation for possible motor neuron disease. Her primary complaint was "hesitancy in speech and low volume."

BRIEF HISTORY OF CASE

The patient, Mrs. M., was a pleasant, well-groomed, and cooperative woman in no acute distress. She was right-handed, had completed tenth grade, was married, and had worked as a florist until her illness. Her problem began approximately 18 months earlier when she experienced a "stroke-like" episode involving right-sided weakness and speech difficulty. According to the patient and her family, the weakness had resolved. Speech, in contrast, seemed to be getting worse. She complained, "I can't form words . . . I know what I'm going to say but I have problems saying it." When asked about word-finding difficulty, she reported that this involved only a confusion of the words *yes* and *no*. When reading, she complained "my eyes flutter and get crossed." Formerly a good speller, she noticed significant problems with writing. She also admitted slowness in *thinking*. She was socially appropriate and had good insight. Though her husband noted problems with speech only, her son described some memory disturbances. She was able to perform her normal activities of daily living, but had withdrawn from outside social contacts.

Past medical history was significant for hypertension, successfully treated since 1983. She had no history of stroke or other systemic disease. She did not drink and had quit smoking 10 years earlier. She had no complaint of visual or hearing changes, weakness in her extremities, or difficulty swallowing. She had no seizures or headaches.

TESTING

THE NEUROLOGICAL EXAMINATION

Mrs. M. was alert, oriented, and cooperative. Remote memory was intact, and she was conversant about current events. Recent memory was adequate, as she was able to recall two of three objects after five minutes. Immediate memory was five digits forward and four backwards. There were several errors on basic calculation tasks. She was unable to abstract any proverbs. Speech was dysarthric and paraphasic.

Physical examination showed normal strength; there was neither atrophy nor fasciculation. Cranial nerves were intact. Sensory examination was intact to touch, pin, and position sense. Coordination examination was normal except for mild dysdiadochokinesis on the left.

A series of diagnostic tests was obtained to rule out treatable causes. A tensilon test was normal. Other tests showed normal thyroid function studies, B^{12}, sedimentation rate, electrolytes, as well as normal renal and liver functions. The brain CT scan results from the local hospital reportedly showed evidence of cerebellar atrophy, but there was no further mention of this. A magnetic resonance imaging study was normal. The electroencephalography (EEG) was normal; there was no epileptiform activity or other abnormality. An electromyographic (EMG) study was normal; there was no evidence of a neuropathic process in arms, legs, or bulbar muscles.

In summary, the patient had a history of controlled hypertension, an essentially normal neurological examination, unconfirmed cerebellar atrophy by CT scan, and a normal magnetic resonance image of the brain. There was a questionable decline of memory and abstraction ability, and a definite complaint of "hesitancy in speech and low volume" that was progressive. Further testing was then undertaken.

THE SPEECH–LANGUAGE EVALUATION

The speech–language evaluation included:

- The Western Aphasia Battery (WAB) (Kertesz, 1982) (Table 18-1)
- Tests of oral, limb, and verbal apraxia
- An oral–facial examination, and speech systems evaluation, supplemented by an instrumental speech analysis (Visi-Pitch Model 6097, interfaced with an IBM XT personal computer).

SPONTANEOUS SPEECH

Background information questions were answered accurately. Mrs. M. was oriented in all spheres and content of speech was appropriate. Errors occurred on items involving numerals (her age, zip code, and telephone number). When describing the "picnic scene" from the WAB, she was complete but hesitant. Grammatical form was somewhat stereotyped (i.e., pronoun + verb + ing), but not agrammatical. She consistently offered pronouns rather than substantive subject nouns (e.g., "They're having a picnic, and he's flying a kite . . . she's drinking and he's eating . . . "). No frank semantic errors occurred.

AUDITORY COMPREHENSION

Mrs. M. answered 20 of 20 yes/no questions, but frequently self-corrected contradictory verbal and nonverbal responses (i.e., shaking her head as she said "yes"). When asked to point to visual stimuli representing a variety of semantic categories, she performed promptly and without error. These

TABLE 18-1.
Performance on the Western Aphasia Battery.

Subtest	Maximum Score	Actual Score
Speech Content	10.0	9.0
Speech Fluency	10.0	6.0
Comprehension	10.0	10.0
Repetition	10.0	8.8
Naming	10.0	8.9
Aphasia Quotient	100.0	85.4
Reading	100.0	83.0
Writing	100.0	66.5
Language Quotient*	100.0	82.6

*Shewan, 1986

categories included objects, forms, letters, numbers, colors, furniture, body parts, finger names, and right/left commands. She performed similarly well on the sequential commands subtest.

REPETITION

On oral repetition of sentences, she achieved a score of 88 of 100 points. This analysis ignored speech sound distortions, accounting only for sound substitutions and word errors. She showed an occasional initial sound repetition, a final sound repetition, one sound intrusion, and one anticipatory error (e.g., s-p-percent). The errors were quite subtle, but suggested some difficulty in sound sequencing.

NAMING

She named 19 of 20 familiar objects on visual confrontation. Her single error was "staple" for paper clip. On a one-minute word fluency task (animal naming) she achieved 12, which is below normal of 18 or better. She was able to complete sentences and respond to questions designed to elicit familiar vocabulary.

READING

Comprehension of single words was intact. On sentence reading, she achieved 10 of 10 for oral reading, and 9 of 10 for comprehension. The error involved confusion of a numerical concept. Additional sentence and short paragraph reading was somewhat slow, with 6 of 8 items correct. She recognized orally spelled words (e.g., hammer, telephone). When asked to spell aloud, she erred on 2 of 6 (e.g., "plncel"/pencil; "gornment"/government).

WRITING

She wrote her name correctly, but her address was incomplete. In response to a picture, writing was slow, and spelling errors were prominent. Whereas she was able to write short, familiar words (e.g., tree, house, man, book), she had frank misspellings on more difficult words (e.g., "balkin"/blanket, "flge"/flag). Additional errors occurred on dictation: "watche"/watch, "teonphone"/telephone, "scruedive"/screwdriver, "hosptil"/hospital. On the writing sentences to dictation task, she wrote: "The quck bown fox juphm over the lazy dog"/The quick brown fox jumped over the lazy dog. Thus, numerous types of errors were noted: letter omissions, phonetically related substitutions, and errors of sequencing.

THE PRAXIS EVALUATION

ORAL AND LIMB PRAXIS

Buccofacial apraxia was normal, as exemplified by her ability to perform, in response to oral command, such tasks as blow, hum, cough, sigh, sniff, puff cheeks, and protrude tongue. Symbolic gestures (e.g., salute, wave goodbye) were slow but otherwise correct. Pretended object uses showed two instances of "body-part-as-object" (BPO). For example, when asked to pretend to light a cigarette, she put her finger in her mouth.

THE SPEECH EVALUATION

Thus far we have described a patient with mild aphasia, mild alexia, and moderate agraphia. She showed intact buccofacial praxis, with mildly impaired limb praxis. We now describe this patient's speech quality.

RESPIRATION

She was able to sniff and pant briskly. Loudness range on discrete tasks was adequate, with good control. Habitual loudness in conversational speech, however, was mildly low overall.

PHONATION

Voice quality was notable for intermittent voice stoppages, poor pitch control (Figure 18-1), and intermittent harshness with increasing roughness towards the end of phrases (Figure 18-2).

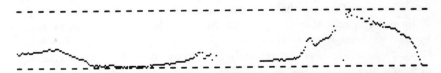

Figure 18-1. Poor pitch control on the discrete vocalization task (/a/) is illustrated. Using the Visi-Pitch (Model 6097), this trace was made showing high to low pitch slide (left) and low to high pitch slide (right). Low end of pitch range (lower horizontal cursor) is 144 Hz; high end of pitch range (upper cursor) is 326 Hz.

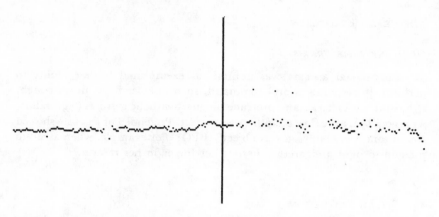

Figure 18–2. Fundamental frequency of prolonged /a/ is shown, illustrating disintegration of voice quality over the length of the sustained sound. The average fundamental frequency for this 8.4 second sample is 181 Hz. The pitch perturbation for the total sample is 0.77 percent; for the first half, 0.65 percent; for the second half, 0.94 percent.

RESONANCE

Oral–nasal resonance balance was within normal limits in conversational speech as well as during cul-de-sac testing.

ARTICULATION

In spontaneous speech, consonants and vowels (especially diphthongs) were distorted, and final consonants were omitted in longer sequences. Articulatory precision was best for sounds in isolation and on automatic speech tasks (e.g., counting), with deterioration in more complex phoneme sequences. As illustrated below, additive phoneme substitutions, intrusive "uh," and effortful intersyllabic transitions compromised phonemic accuracy.

To assess articulation further, Mrs. M. was asked to repeat polysyllabic words five times in succession. She repeated some words (e.g., snowball, vegetable) without error or variability on repeated trials. Some variability occurred on *refrigerator* ("refriger-wator . . . re-riguh . . . "), and *valuable* ("val-ble . . . valuhble . . . "). The difficult item *catastrophe* was quite variable, as follows: "kuh-tas-uh-suh . . . kuh-tas-ter-feef . . . kuh-tras-uh-ee . . . kuh-tras-truh-kuh-tas-uh." These productions show sound additions and sequencing errors and variability on repeated trials.

DIADOCHOKINETIC RATES

Single syllables /p/, /t/ and /k/ were initiated hesitantly, but thereafter produced rapidly and evenly (Figure 18-3). In contrast, the syllable sequence /p-t-k/ and words (e.g., puppy) were sequenced slowly and effortfully.

PROSODY

During automatic speech (counting) and rapid repetition of single syllables, her rate was within normal limits. In conversational speech and sentence repetition, her rate was slow overall due to sound prolongation, and intersyllabic pause (syllable segregation). Stress was equalized and pitch contour was flattened. Overall, the rhythmic quality of speech was lost.

In summary, our patient presented a motor speech disorder with moderately impaired intelligibility overall. Dysphonia and dysprosody were perceptually prominent, while articulatory imprecision was secondary. Voice stoppages contributed to equalization of stress and segregation of syllables. The perceptual and instrumental results were consistent with diagnoses of dysarthria (prominent dysphonia) and apraxia of speech (phonemic and syllabic selection and sequencing difficulty). The perceptually prominent dysprosody—halting speech, phoneme prolongations, syllable segregation, and flattened stress/pitch contour—shares features of both ataxic dysarthria and apraxia of speech (Kent & Rosenbek, 1982, 1983).

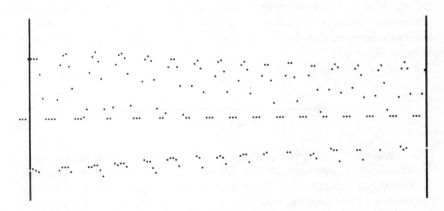

Figure 18-3. Alternate motion rate (AMR) for the syllable /t/ is illustrated. The top trace is the intensity of the signal and the bottom trarce is the pitch. The patient repeated 17 syllables in 4.1 seconds for an AMR of 4.1 syllables per second. Following voice/articulatory initiation difficulty (not shown) diadochokinesis was rapid and even.

NEUROPSYCHOLOGICAL EVALUATION

A complete neuropsychological evaluation was conducted. The results will be highlighted here. On the Wechsler Adult Intelligence Scale-Revised (Wechsler, 1981) she achieved verbal, performance, and full scale intelligence quotients of 80, 87, and 82, respectively. This performance was within the low-normal range, a level roughly commensurate with her attained educational and vocational level. In contrast, memory function testing revealed significant memory losses bilaterally, with semantic memory performance ranging from moderate to severe and figural memory performance from mild to moderate. Retrieval was somewhat better than recall for both areas. Timed tests of higher cognitive functions revealed slow processing, and diminished problem solving and adaptive functioning. There were no indications of constructional apraxia.

Thus, higher cortical functions were impaired beyond that to be expected of the normal aging process. Deficiencies were of a general nature; there were no lateralizing or localizing features. Loss in adaptive functioning and memory did not appear to be a function of her significant communication difficulty. In summary, the consulting neuropsychologist concluded that this patient's profile was compatible with the typical effects of an early dementing process.

One year later, a follow-up neuropsychological evaluation was attempted. At this time, speech was "unintelligible, even with single words in context." Testing was limited to nonverbal items. Results were interpreted to represent a significant "across the board" decline in general mental functioning. Mrs. M. continued to remain isolated at home. The family recounted occasional instances of disinhibition (hostility) by the patient. A mild to moderate level of depression was ascertained by history and by clinical examination.

DISCUSSION

When seen by Speech-Language Pathology in the early months of 1986, the clinical diagnoses were aphasia, alexia, agraphia, limb apraxia, as well as apraxia of speech and dysarthria, with prominent dysphonia and dysprosody. We wondered, Is this a focal aphasia-apraxia syndrome secondary to a left hemisphere stroke? Could the dysarthria be explained by possible cerebellar atrophy? Was this a slowly progressive aphasia without generalized dementia (Duffy, 1987; Mesulam, 1982; Wechsler, 1977; Wechsler et al, 1982)? Was this an atypical Alzheimer's disease with spasticity and ataxia (e.g., Aikawa, Suzuki, Iwasaki, & Iizuka, 1985)? Or, was this a mixed cortical–subcortical dementing illness (Albert, 1978; Cummings, 1985)? Table 18-2 summarizes the results of the evaluation.

CONCLUSION

The thorough medical evaluation ruled out other disorders potentially associated with speech–language and cognitive impairment. The neuropsychological evaluations documented progressive cognitive decline. The speech–language pathology evaluation characterized the neurogenic

TABLE 18-2.
Clinical features of a woman with early dementia of unknown type consistent with cortical or subcortical disease.*

	Subcortical	Cortical
Mental Status		
Language		Aphasia, alexia, agraphia.
Memory		Semantic and figural memory loss, mild-severe.
Higher cognitive	Slowness, reduced adaptive functioning.	(Fund of information good; proverbs poor; acalculia present.)
Personality/Mood	Appropriate at 18 months; disinhibited with some hostility at 36 months in association with mild to moderate depression.	
Motor System		
Speech	Dysprosody** Dysarthria with dysphonia prominent.	Dysprosody** Apraxia of speech†
Posture		Normal
Gait		Normal
Motor speed	Mild dysdiadochokinesis	
Movement	Normal	Normal

*Dimensions important for distinguishing cortical–subcortical dementias adapted from Cummings, 1985; Cummings & Benson, 1984, 1986.
**Dysprosodic features consistent with ataxic dysarthria and apraxia of speech (Kent & Rosenbek, 1982).
†Kent & Rosenbek, 1983.

communication disorder, but the anatomy and mechanism of the aphasic-apraxic-dysarthric complex remained unclear. The final diagnosis was "early dementia of unknown type." We suggest that this neurobehavioral profile was consistent with a cortical–subcortical neuropathology.

Although this diagnostic puzzle remained unresolved, this case provides the opportunity to highlight some current clinical issues. First, aphasia is now recognized as an important diagnostic feature of dementia of the Alzheimer type (Cummings, Benson, Hill, & Read, 1986), but precisely how Alzheimer's aphasia differs from the language of stroke-related dementia (Hier, Hagenlocker, & Shindler, 1985; Nicholas, Obler, Albert, & Helm-Estabrooks, 1985) or other syndromes (Helm-Estabrooks, Nicholas and Morgan, Chapter 20, this volume) is not yet clear. Second, aphasia (or apraxia or agnosia) may appear as the sole or prominent feature of a dementing illness, usually Alzheimer's or Pick's disease (DeRenzi, 1986; Holland, McBurney, Moossy, & Reinmuth, 1985). Third, early or prominent aphasia in dementing illness may present in younger patients (Chui, Teng, Henderson, & Moy, 1985) or herald rapid decline (Kaszniak, Fox, Gandell, Garron, Huckman, & Ramsey, 1978).

Thus, three challenges for future research are (1) to identify the distinguishing features of aphasia in focal disease versus aphasia in diffuse, dementing illnesses, (2) to determine the localizing value of dysarthria or apraxia co-occurring with dementia, and (3) to understand the prognostic significance of aphasia as a prominent manifestation of a dementing illness. The further study of the differences among focal versus diffuse, and reversible versus progressive syndromes *in terms of speech and language characteristics* (Hier et al., 1985; Horner, 1985; Horner, Lathrop, Fish, Dawson, 1987; Kirschner, Webb, Kelly, & Wells, 1984; Nicholas et al., 1985) may help solve similar diagnostic dilemmas in the future. The interdisciplinary, comprehensive evaluation of such challenging diagnostic cases may ultimately enhance our diagnostic precision.

ACKNOWLEDGMENTS

James M. Gilchrist, M.D., Department of Medicine, Division of Neurology, Duke University Medical Center.

Patrick E. Logue, Ph.D., Division of Medical Psychology, Department of Psychiatry, Duke University Medical Center.

REFERENCES

Aikawa, H., Suzuki, K., Iwasaki, Y., & Iizuka, R. (1985). Atypical Alzheimer's disease with spastic paresis and ataxia. *Annals of Neurology, 17,* 297–300.

Albert, M.L. (1978). Subcortical dementia. In R. Katzman, R.D. Terry, & K.L. Bick (Eds.), *Alzheimer's disease: Senile dementia and related disorders (Aging, Vol. 7)*. New York: Raven Press.

Chui, H.C., Teng, E.L., Henderson, V.W., & Moy, A.C. (1985). Clinical subtypes of dementia of the Alzheimer type. *Neurology, 35*, 1544-1550.

Cummings, J.L. (1985). *Clinical neuropsychiatry*. Orlando, FL: Grune & Stratton.

Cummings, J.L., & Benson, D.F. (1984). Subcortical dementia, review of an emerging concept. *Archives of Neurology, 41*, 874-879.

Cummings, J.L., & Benson, D.F. (1986). Dementia of the Alzheimer type, an inventory of diagnostic clinical features. *Journal of the American Geriatric Society, 34*, 12-19.

Cummings, J.L., Benson, D.F., Hill, M.A., & Read, S. (1986). Aphasia in dementia of the Alzheimer type. *Neurology, 35*, 394-397.

DeRenzi, E. (1986). Slowly progressive visual agnosia or apraxia without dementia. *Cortex, 22*, 171-180.

Duffy, J.R. (1987). Slowly progressive aphasia. In R.H. Brookshire (Ed.), *Clinical aphasiology conference, Volume 17*. Minneapolis: BRK Publishers.

Hier, D.B., Hagenlocker, K., & Shindler, A.G. (1985). Language disintegration in dementia: Effects of etiology and severity. *Brain and Language, 25*, 117-133.

Holland, A.L., McBurney, D.H., Moossy, J., & Reinmuth, O.M. (1985). The dissolution of language in Pick's disease with neurofibrillary tangles: A case study. *Brain and Language, 24*, 36-58.

Horner, J. (1985). Language disorders associated with Alzheimer's dementia, left hemisphere stroke, and progressive illness of uncertain etiology. In R.H. Brookshire (Ed.), *Clinical aphasiology conference, Volume 15*. Minneapolis: BRK Publishers.

Horner, J., Lathrop, D.L., Fish, A.G., & Dawson, D. (1987). Agraphia in left and right hemisphere stroke and Alzheimer dementia patients. In R.H. Brookshire (Ed.), *Clinical aphasiology conference, Volume 17*. Minneapolis: BRK Publishers.

Kaszniak, A.W., Fox, J., Gandell, D.L., Garron, D.C., Huckman, M.S., & Ramsey, R.G. (1978). Predictors of mortality in presenile and senile dementia. *Annals of Neurology, 3*, 246-252.

Kent, R.D., & Rosenbek, J.C. (1982). Prosodic disturbance and neurologic lesion. *Brain and Language, 15*, 259-291.

Kent, R.D., & Rosenbek, J.C. (1983). Acoustic patterns of apraxia of speech. *Journal of Speech and Hearing Research, 26*, 231-248.

Kertesz, A. (1982). *Western aphasia battery*. New York: Grune & Stratton.

Mesulam, M-M. (1982). Slowly progressive aphasia without generalized dementia. *Annals of Neurology, 11*, 592-598.

Nicholas, M., Obler, L.K., Albert, M.L., & Helm-Estabrooks, N. (1985). Empty speech in Alzheimer's disease and fluent aphasia. *Journal of Speech and Hearing Research, 28*, 405-410.

Shewan, C. (1986). The language quotient (LQ): A new measure for the Western Aphasia Battery. *Journal of Communication Disorders, 19*, 427-439.

Wechsler, A.F. (1977). Presenile dementia presenting as aphasias. *Journal of*

Neurology, Neurosurgery, and Psychiatry, 40, 303–305.

Wechsler, A.F., Verity, M.A., Rosenschein, S., Fried, I., & Scheibel, A.B. (1982). Pick's disease: A clinical, computed tomographic, and histologic study with Golgi impregnation observations. *Archives of Neurology, 39,* 287–290.

Wechsler, D. (1981). *Wechsler Adult Intelligence Scale-Revised Manual.* New York: The Psychological Corporation.

CHAPTER 19

AUDREY L. HOLLAND

DIAGNOSING PICK'S
DISEASE: THE UTILITY
OF CLINICAL PROBLEM
SOLVING

*M*r. E., the patient discussed in this chapter, has been described in detail elsewhere (Holland et al., 1985). This current presentation is motivated by an attempt to describe the problem-solving behavior that occurred in relation to this case. As the reader will see, much time has passed between initially meeting the patient and the writing of this chapter. In the interim, a relevant literature has emerged that is useful in explaining Mr. E.'s problem. Nevertheless, Mr. E. and others like him remain diagnostically challenging, and demand thoughtful problem-solving attempts.

INITIAL INTERACTIONS WITH MR. E.

My involvement with this patient began when I was casually asked by an acquaintance if I might be interested in trying to provide some management ideas for his 76-year-old father, Mr. E. My friend told me that his father had had a stroke and "couldn't understand anything said to him." The son reported that Mr. E. "also could not talk." Having made the assumption that the man had global aphasia, I became even more interested when the son added, "My dad can read and write very well, and he conducts all of his personal and business affairs through reading and writing." A double dissociation of language modalities would have been unique in my experience, and the possibility that such was the case made Mr. E. even more interesting to me. The son asked me to visit Mr. E., provided his father agreed to it.

I had already planned my approach to the family as I neared the end of my drive to the house two days later. It was essentially to convince them that Mr. E., of course, had reading and writing deficits consonant with my predetermined diagnosis of global aphasia, to arrange for formal testing, subsequent direct therapy, and to plan counseling for the family. I was greeted at the door by a dapper, physically fit, elderly gentleman, just returned from his daily three-mile bike ride. Mr. E. gave me his calling card, with the following additional message:

Hearing is good physically
Language sounds — not sense — noise

Figure 19-1 is a fragment of our first "conversation." It was conducted in silence, or at least in as complete a silence as I could manage, and Mr. E. frequently shoved the card in front of me as a reminder. Insofar as formal conversational parameters can have written analogs, such as well-timed turn taking and rapid information exchange, this was a normally structured interaction. The information included in Figure 19-1, as well as additional information he provided, was correct. This extremely good recall of the events of his own life was taken as evidence of intact episodic memory. Although the 90 minute visit was polite and pleasant, Mr. E. was very serious throughout it. He did not smile or laugh at all and was generally emotionally unresponsive.

It should be noted that the events just described occurred in 1978. At that time most of us knew how to differentiate among motor speech disorders as a function of underlying neurological conditions. However, the burst of information that is currently allowing speech–language pathologists to make similar distinctions among patterns of language deficits that accompany various neurogenic conditions had not yet really begun. For example, texts like Bayles and Kaszniak (1987) were simply not available at that time, and with the exception of aphasia, careful descriptions of neurogenic language disorders were just beginning to emerge. I had never seen a patient like Mr. E. I did not know what was wrong with him; I needed much more information. I did not know what to recommend to him or to his family that might be of help to them. Mr. E. did not seem to be "aphasic" in any conventional sense.

A critical aspect of diagnostic decision making concerns one's ability to recognize what one does and does not know. Once recognized, this sort of ignorance must be admitted. This is not always easy to do. However, I had never seen a person with such extensive dissociations and it was fairly easy to come to grips with my own inexperience.

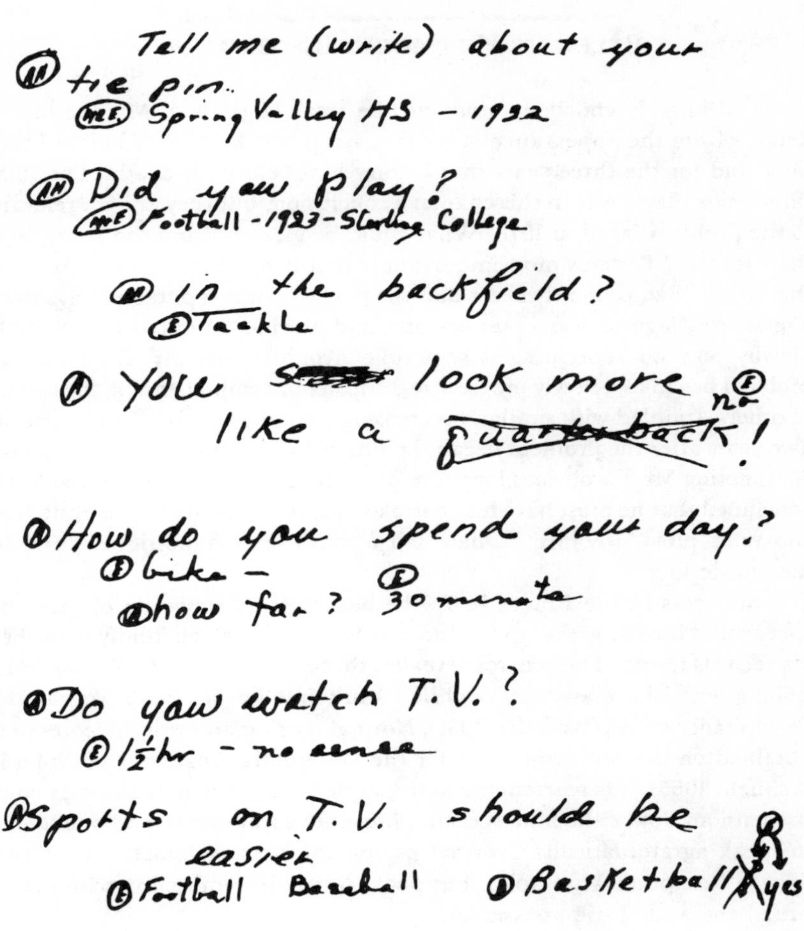

Figure 19-1. Fragment of my first "conversation" with Mr. E.

The obvious and natural next step should have been extensive formal evaluation, not only of Mr. E.'s language, but of his overall neuropsychological functioning. However, although Mr. E. tolerated me rather gracefully, he made it clear that he was not interested in extensive formal diagnostic testing. With that avenue closed, two other approaches became more appealing. The first was to rely heavily on the family's excellent ability to recall Mr. E.'s recent history, and to look for more complete evidence concerning the extent of his reading comprehension ability. The second was then to relate this history to the available literature. Both approaches were used.

RELEVANT HISTORICAL INFORMATION

I ultimately ended up studying the final 12 years of Mr. E.'s life in detail—from the appearance of his first symptoms nine years before I met him, and for the three years that I knew him before his death. The final three years play a role in this chapter's conclusion, but they are not relevant to the problem faced in 1978. What could be gleaned from the family and their records? Perhaps most important is that it became increasingly clear that Mr. E. had probably never had the stroke he was reputed to have had. The stroke diagnosis was a post hoc one, and provides an instructive example of why post hoc reasoning is sometimes troublesome. Mr. E.'s language problem began as a slowly progressive difficulty in comprehending the speech of others, coupled with similarly increasing paraphasic errors in his speech. Two years after the problem began, he finally saw a neurologist. This physician, noting Mr. E.'s obvious language problem, as well as an abnormal EEG, concluded that he must have had a stroke that otherwise had gone unnoticed two years previously. Mr. E. had had a stroke by diagnostic fiat, not by diagnostic fact.

Six years before I met Mr. E., he had received six weeks of intensive speech and language therapy at Indiana University, which kindly furnished his records to me. The records revealed that at that time Mr. E. was functioning with above-average Wechsler Adult Intelligence Scale Verbal and Performance scores (Wechsler, 1981). Normal reading and writing scores were obtained on the Minnesota Test for the Differential Diagnosis of Aphasia (Schuell, 1965). These strengths were coupled with impaired auditory comprehension, slow, deliberate speech, phonemic paraphasias, and a tendency to speak agrammatically. Normal peripheral hearing bilaterally, normal Speech Reception Thresholds, but poor speech discrimination scores comprised the audiologic assessment.

The problems Mr. E. demonstrated when I first saw him were similar to these, but in exacerbated form. Steady and gradual deterioration of auditory comprehension and speech production had occurred since his intensive treatment. Within a year after it, Mr. E. had begun relying more and more heavily on writing to communicate, and consistently requested others to write to him because written messages were easier for him to understand. He stopped speaking altogether in 1974 and he lost his lifelong interest in music at about the same time. His written messages became more fragmentary and somewhat more telegraphic over this period.

When I first saw Mr. E., there was very strong evidence of both his good functional reading comprehension and his moderate writing ability. First, Mr. E. managed all of his own business affairs, including bank accounts and income tax. Second, he continued a lifelong habit of shopping by mail, and as late as 1976, had ordered a grandfather clock kit, which he successfully built by following the written directions, over the course of a year. He maintained a vast correspondence with friends and relatives across the country, saving copies of all of his own letters. This written record attested not only to his reading and writing skills, but to his memory as well. His family felt that his hearing sensitivity seemed to be functionally intact; however, sounds were sources of annoyance to him, rather than sources of information. To be sure, there was increased deterioration of written communication, but it was much more evident in grammar than in lexicon. Figure 19-2 is a characteristic letter that Mr. E. typed and sent to friends and relatives. The content of his letter suggested both good semantic and episodic memory. I have added the handwritten explanatory notes that appear on the figure.

SEARCHING THE LITERATURE

With the above information as the background, the medical and neurolinguistic literature was searched. The most pertinent problem to study was pure-word deafness. Of particular concern was whether there was a literature suggesting that this disorder could be manifested as a progressive condition. I could not find corroborating evidence. A second question was to determine what sorts of progressive disorders produce mutism over their courses. There was a sparse literature suggesting that mutism was associated with dementing conditions. However, this literature also suggested that mutism usually occurred late in dementia, when semantic–lexical, cognitive, and memory deficits were well advanced. This contrasted sharply with Mr. E., who was filing his income tax, doing his shopping by mail, and maintaining his correspondence, going to church, and being neat and courteous. Mr. E.'s problem was simply not well described in the available literature at the time I first saw him.

THE CLINICIAN'S ROLE WITH UNUSUAL CASES

The clinician who sees patients who have rare or unexplained disorders has two professional responsibilities. The first is to the patient and the family; the second is to the profession, for the rare case is likely to add to our knowledge base. With respect to clinical management, some attempt must be made to help such patients by seeking other consultations, not only from other professionals, but from colleagues in other professions as well. Undertaking some trial treatment is probably also in order, provided that it is

Dear Robert, Ruth and Family:

I cannot compose the letter, not speak, hearing is good,
language sounds, not sense, noise. Stroke.

Donald and Joan from 2563 Meinert Road to Fredric and Faith
for 8066 Oxbridge Drive. Furniture for room, desk, typewriter,
TV, closet, bed, and pictures on the walls.   *] moved from D-J (Meinert Rd) to F+F (Oxbridge Drive)*

THANKSGIVING DINNER -- Oxbridge

    Wendell, Jean, Cynthia, Willson, Laurie.

    Donald, Joan, Ann, Ruth, Elaine, Susan.   *] accurate list of dinner guests*

    Fred, Faith, Benjy, Joel, Will.

    Russell and Rhoda * , and Aunt Rose

    Cousin music piano, cello, flute, and anyones turned. — *after-dinner tradition*
    Ann -- H. S. Band, Benjy -- Orchestra.

    Cousin Slumbing Party tonight living room CWL, ARES, and BJW.- *initials refer to cousins. Typical of pre-illness style*

    Friday -- Duquesne Trolley afternoon. Pictures for their
anyones.

Tuesday afternoon Waldo and Vernice to Oxbridge tonight. The
pictures to have Marian monument Quinter Cemetery. W and V seen
clock 1976 make, Totem Pole 1977 make to Benjy.   *] W + V brought pictures of M's monument.*

Monday evening for R. P. Home directors, Wilbur McElroy and
daughter, Topeka, to Kenya this week. Wilbur seen clock and
Totem Pole.

Kind of lovings.

        Sincerely,

Figure 19-2. Example of a letter sent to friends and relatives.

carefully explained and justified only as a trial. These courses were followed.
Mr. E. was informally assessed by other speech–language pathologists, and
by a neuropsychologist. He permitted a neurological evaluation to be completed by a neurologist. These professionals all were as baffled as I was by
Mr. E.'s particular constellation of strengths and weaknesses. Trial therapy
intended to help Mr. E. and his family communicate more quickly and easily
consisted of training in Amerind Sign. Mr. E. accommodatingly learned 50
signs, which he never used spontaneously at home or in the clinic. He continued to prefer writing his notes. He quit therapy when he received the
first bill for this "help."

    I still saw Mr. E. and his family informally. At my request, the family
began taking notes on his behavior. His reading and writing skills deteriorated
over the next two years with an accelerating course. Behavioral problems
began to occur, and grew more serious. For example, Mr. E. began riding
his bicycle at top speed across major highways, rather than cautiously riding
around his neighborhood for exercise, as he had when I first met him. But

even though his reading and writing were worsening, his letter and note writing continued. Figure 19-3 is the last letter Mr. E. is known to have written.

Mr. E. was finally placed in a nursing home when his behavior became unmanageable at home. I asked the family to save his correspondence, which is the source of the letters included above. I also asked them to consider an autopsy in the event of Mr. E.'s death. In 1980, Mr. E. died of respiratory illness. The neuropathology report indicated that his language disorder was the result of Pick's disease. I began piecing the family's records and Mr. E.'s own record of his disorder together.

CONCLUDING THOUGHTS

When Mr. E.'s story was published after his death, it became part of a newly emerging literature describing the variety of language disorders that occur in dementia. (Other examples include Cummings and Duchen, 1981; Kirshner et al., 1984; Obler & Albert, 1981; and Wechsler, 1977) This recent literature suggests that language and memory deterioration in the various dementias can differ distinctively in presentation and in course (Hier et al., 1985; Schwartz, Marin, & Saffran, 1979). Some observers suggest that these patterns and dissociations of language can be used to differentiate some types of dementia early in their course (Bayles & Kaszniak, 1987). It is obvious that the study of dementing language can inform theories of language, brain and behavior. The scientific study of neurolinguistics will be advanced if it is shown that the progressive and irreversible predominantly cortical dementias, such as Pick's and Alzheimer's diseases, multi-infarct dementia, and Kreuzfeld-Jacob, have differing language patterns to accompany their differing underlying pathologies.

Dear Ruth and Bob:

I cannot compose The letter, not speak, language is good, hearing is good, not sense, noise. Stroke 1970.

Note not Mary Jane, and MI Tammy.

Envelope none Roger.

Sincerely,

Figure 19-3. Last letter written by Mr. E.

From the standpoint of the dementing patient, at first glance it might appear that differential diagnosis of incurable diseases such as these is possibly a thankless enterprise. However, there are patient management reasons that make differential diagnosis important. As we learn more about language disorders in the so-called incurable dementias, we may be of increasing help in differentiating them from the reversible ones. Another management reason concerns the similarity of Mr. E.'s language problem to a recently elucidated disorder known as "progressive aphasia" (Kirshner et al., 1987; Mesulam, 1982). Progressive aphasia occurs in the absence of a stroke or other neurological disorder that could explain it. Patients with this slowly progressive language disorder differ from Mr. E. by their failure to develop dementia subsequently. Thus, they have a relatively less gloomy prognosis, and may possibly be helped by appropriate clinical management.

I am presently following at least four other patients whose symptoms are quite similar to Mr. E.'s. At the time of this writing, I feel relatively confident that three of them have Pick's disease, a disorder I didn't even know about in 1978, and the other a progressive aphasia which I only found out about in 1982. For two of the presumed Pick's disease patients and for the presumed progressive aphasia patient, I am following Mr. E.'s lead. I am encouraging them to maintain their reading and writing skills through correspondence, to keep diaries, and to communicate around the house using notes. In the case of one patient who has usable but markedly limited output, I am also encouraging her to use short conversational interchanges that I have devised for her and which she has memorized. I do not believe these activities are merely palliative forms of treatment, regardless of whether the patients ultimately are found to have Pick's disease, progressive aphasia, or still another as yet undescribed disorder.

References

Bayles, K.A., & Kaszniak, A. W. (1987). *Communication and cognition in normal aging and dementia.* San Diego: College-Hill Press.

Cummings, J., & Duchen, L. (1981). Kluver-Bucy syndrome in Pick's disease: Clinical and pathologic correlations. *Neurology, 31*, 1415-1422.

Hier, D.B., Hagenlocker, K., & Schindler, A.G. (1985). Language disintegration in dementia: Effects of etiology and severity. *Brain and Language, 25*, 117-133.

Holland, A.L., McBurney, D.H., Moossy, J., & Reinmuth, O.M. (1985). The dissolution of language in Pick's disease with neurofibrillary tangles: A case study. *Brain and Language, 24*, 36-58.

Kirshner, H.S., Webb, W.G., Kelly, M.P., & Wells, C.E. (1984). Language disturbance: An initial symptom of cortical degeneration and dementia. *Archives of Neurology, 41*, 491-496.

Kirshner, H.S., Tandridag, O., Thurman, L., & Whetsell, W.O. (1987). Progressive aphasia without dementia: Two cases with focal spongiform degeneration. *Annals of Neurology, 22,* 527-532.

Mesulam, M-M. (1982). Slowly progressive aphasia without generalized dementia. *Annals of Neurology, 11,* 592-598.

Obler, L.K., & Albert, M.L. (1981). Language and aging: A neurobehavioral analysis. In D.S. Beasley & G.A. Davis (Eds.), *Aging: Communication processes and disorders.* New York: Grune & Stratton.

Schuell, H. (1965). *The Minnesota test for differential diagnosis of aphasia.* Minneapolis: University of Minnesota Press.

Schwartz, M., Marin, O., & Saffran, E. (1979). Dissociation of language function in dementia: A case study. *Brain and Language, 7,* 277-306.

Wechsler, A.F. (1977). Presenile dementia presenting as aphasia. *Journal of Neurology, Neurosurgery and Psychiatry, 40,* 303-305.

Wechsler, D. (1981). *Wechsler Adult Intelligence Scale-Revised Manual.* New York: The Psychological Corporation.

CHAPTER 20

Nancy Helm-Estabrooks
Marjorie Nicholas
Alisa Morgan

"FIFTY-TWO-YEAR OLD MALE WITH STAMMERING SPEECH — CVA?"

Our Speech–Language Pathology department received a consult from Neurology that stated:

> 52 y-o w male with stammering speech. ? CVA. Please evaluate.

While the consult appeared relatively straightforward, we soon realized that this case presented a significant challenge to our skills as diagnosticians. In the end, we were only able to narrow the etiological choices to the "best guess," but enroute to this tentative diagnosis, several other interesting possibilities presented themselves. These alternative diagnoses were based on the neurological, speech–language, and neuropsychological findings, as well as the patient's history.

BRIEF HISTORY

Mr. P. was a 52-year-old, right-handed, white man who was unmarried until age 47. Although it was somewhat difficult to establish a clear history, the following information was obtained. Mr. P.'s first language was Canadian French, which he spoke exclusively until learning English in grammar school.

When seen by us, he reported that his French was quite "rusty." Mr. P. graduated from high school and entered the armed services, during which time he was stationed in Guam for one year. Following discharge he worked first in a tannery (approximately 12 years) and then in a paper plant (approximately 15 years). According to Mr. P., he lost his job at the paper plant because of cutbacks and subsequently found part-time employment as a security guard for a nursing home.

Mr. P. had a history of severe headaches, treated as migraines, which apparently began shortly after discharge from the armed services. Other medical problems included a poorly defined gastric disorder, angina, hypertension, and a lymphoproliferative disorder. In addition, he reported a gradual, 10-year, unspecified decline in writing skills, which a physician had attributed to Parkinson's disease.

Mr. P. experienced two incidents of sudden speech arrest, at four years and one year prior to admission; while engaged in conversation he went "blank" and "nothing would come out." These incidents lasted for several minutes, with slow return of clear speech over the next 15 minutes. In the year prior to admission, however, there was a gradual deterioration of speech. In addition, he reported that he misplaced items, was confused about travel directions, and had difficulty understanding and responding to questions. Both Mr. P. and his wife suspected hearing problems were the basis of his comprehension difficulties, although his hearing was not tested until he was admitted to our facility.

TESTING

THE NEUROLOGICAL EXAMINATION

The elemental neurological examination was remarkable for a decreased left nasolabial fold, frequent oral–facial dyskinesias, and slowed fast-finger movements bilaterally. An EEG showed intermittent, left temporal slowing. A CT scan performed at the time of admission revealed a questionable small area of low density deep to the supramarginal gyrus in the left hemisphere, a questionable small area of low density in the head of the left caudate, prominent sulci bilaterally, particularly in the frontal lobes and the superior parietal lobule, prominent Sylvian fissures, and enlarged frontal horns bilaterally.

THE SPEECH AND LANGUAGE EVALUATION

In order to determine the nature of Mr. P.'s speech and language problem, our evaluation included the following tests:

- Boston Diagnostic Aphasia Examination (BDAE)
- Informal supplementary language tests of grammatical skills
- Boston Naming Test
- Boston Praxis Examination
- Full audiological evaluation

FIRST IMPRESSIONS

Mr. P. was well-groomed, pleasant, socially appropriate, and cooperative throughout testing, although he appeared tense and anxious. He became slightly tearful when first asked about the speech problems, but he did not show signs of emotional lability. Myoclonic-type movements occasionally were noted around the eyes and in the shoulder area during both speech and some nonspeech activities. He tried to control the shoulder movements by crossing his arms and holding them against his chest.

SPEECH–LANGUAGE TEST RESULTS

GENERAL TEST BEHAVIOR

During informal conversation, Mr. P.'s most obvious difficulty was in verbal expression. Formal testing, however, quickly revealed a more serious side to his disorder. He had great difficulty establishing, maintaining, and switching set. Occasionally, he would stare into space, making no response until the examiner refocused his attention and reestablished set. This was particularly evident on subtests of auditory and reading comprehension. In addition, Mr. P. often asked for repetition of stimulus items or instructions, giving the impression of a hearing problem.

CONVERSATIONAL SPEECH

Mr. P.'s conversational speech was characterized by a French-Canadian accent, slow rate, hypophonia, occasional palilalic repetition of phrases, and stuttering, manifested by severe blocks and multiple syllable and word repetitions. Many attempts to speak were accompanied by tremors or clonic-like movements of the oral musculature. All of these features contributed to relatively short utterance length and a limited range of grammatical constructions. Melodic line was within normal limits for short utterances, but became restricted as severity of blocks and repetitions increased. Paraphasias were rare. Overall, he earned an Aphasia Severity Rating (ASR) of 2 on the BDAE, indicating that his speech difficulties resulted in frequent failures to convey information without help from the listener (see Figure 20-1 for Mr. P.'s BDAE Severity Rating and Speech Profile). A transcription of his

Boston Diagnostic Aphasia Examination

Patient's Name ____ Mr. P. _____ Date of rating _____

Rated by _____

APHASIA SEVERITY RATING SCALE

0. No usable speech or auditory comprehension.

1. All communication is through fragmentary expression; great need for inference, questioning, and guessing by the listener. The range of information that can be exchanged is limited, and the listener carries the burden of communication.

2. Conversation about familiar subjects is possible with help from the listener. There are frequent failures to convey the idea, but patient shares the burden of communication with the examiner.

3. The patient can discuss <u>almost all everyday problems</u> with little or no assistance. Reduction of speech and/or comprehension, however, makes conversation about certain material difficult or impossible.

4. Some obvious loss of fluency in speech or facility of comprehension, without significant limitation on ideas expressed or form of expression.

5. Minimal discernible speech handicaps; patient may have subjective difficulties that are not apparent to listener.

RATING SCALE PROFILE OF SPEECH CHARACTERISTICS

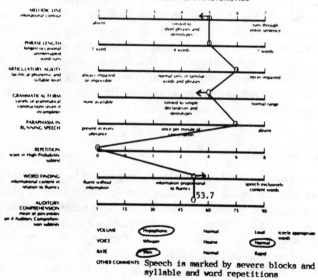

Figure 20-1. Results of Mr. P.'s Boston Diagnostic Aphasia Examination.

verbal Cookie Theft Picture description is included in Figure 20-2. Occasionally he was able to convey a message he could not articulate by writing words.

AUDITORY COMPREHENSION

Set and attentional problems as well as confusion interfered with auditory comprehension testing. Mr. P. performed in the fifty-third percentile overall on the BDAE auditory comprehension subtests, with his best scores on word discrimination and body-part identification. Performance deteriorated as test items became longer and more complex. In the subtest of complex ideational material, he tended toward indiscriminant streaks of affirmative or negative responses. Supplementary language testing showed poor comprehension of passives, possessives, and verb complements.

VERBAL REPETITION AND NAMING

Oral repetition was restricted to reproduction of some single words and 1 of 16 sentences. He had great difficulty initiating repetition responses, and when he was able to initiate a repetition, he often rephrased the item; for

```
WELL.... THE WO-WOMANAN IS IS IS WASHING THE THE D-DISHES.
THE KID IS   IS GETTING THE COOKIES.   AND THE GIRL (GUY?)
IS - I THINK HIS HIS GONNA HE'S GONNA (LIAS?) TO TO....
WELL, I'LL GO I"LL GO TO THE THE THE GIRL.  SHE, YOU, SHE
WANTS  SHE WANTS  SHE WANTS THE COOKIE.   AND UM.... THE
WATER IS   IS..........HMM...........


EXAMINER: CAN"T YOU FIND THE WORDS OR ARE YOU JUST HAVING
A HARD TIME SAYING THEM?   DO YOU HAVE THE WORDS FOR WHAT"S
HAPPENING THERE?


YES, YES........HE GOT.... THE SI-SINK IS IS IS OVERFA-FA
FLOW.... TO THE ......
```

Figure 20-2. Mr. P.'s verbal description of the Cookie Theft Picture.

example, "I came, I came to . . . to home," for *I got home from work*. Responsive naming (24/30) and confrontation naming (97/115) were areas of relative strength on the BDAE. On the Boston Naming Test (BNT), however, Mr. P. correctly named only 22 of 60 pictured objects and was not helped by phonemic cues.

READING AND WRITING

Oral reading was very good if one overlooked dysfluencies (10/10 words; 9/10 sentences). Performance on reading comprehension subtests, however, was reminiscent of that for auditory comprehension. Set and attentional problems were evident and performance deteriorated as items became more complex. Once in set, he earned 9/10 points on word–picture matching, but only 5/10 for sentences and paragraphs.

Mr. P. produced generally legible cursive writing. Writing was markedly slow (for example, he took over 3 minutes to write only 13 letters of the alphabet), and he often abandoned attempts at spelling words. His written description of the Cookie Theft Picture (see Figure 20-3) contained unfinished sentences with no capitalization, and empty, prepositional phrases for example, "to cookies to him and is to his".

AUTOMATIZED SPEECH AND VERBAL/NONVERBAL AGILITY

In producing automatized sequences, Mr. P. performed best in counting to 21. He recited the days of the week with long pauses, but produced only seven consecutive letters of the alphabet and five consecutive months of the year. He was unable to recite any nursery rhymes, stating that he did not remember the words. He could not sing or tap rhythmic patterns. Both verbal (3/8) and nonverbal (4/10) agility were impaired. Tongue movements and production of multisyllabic words were particularly difficult.

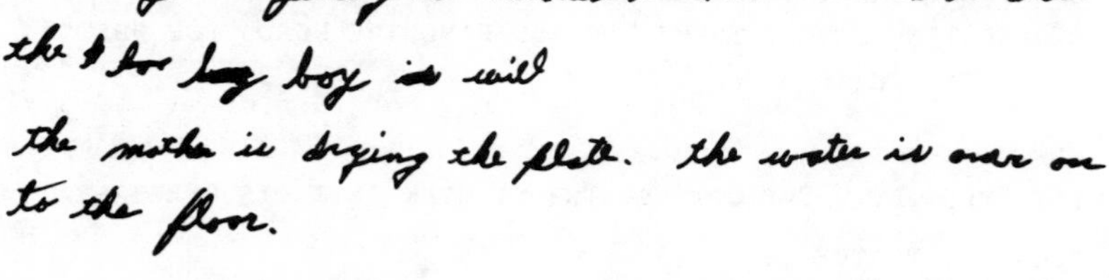

Figure 20-3. Mr. P.'s written description of the Cookie Theft Picture.

PRAXIS TESTING

Testing with the Boston Praxis Exam showed a mild transitive limb apraxia (gestures with implied use of object; e.g., combing hair), and a mild finger apraxia (e.g., thumbing a ride). Performance improved on imitation. There was no evidence of buccofacial apraxia.

AUDIOLOGICAL TESTING

The results of the audiological evaluation showed that pure-tone air and bone conduction thresholds were within normal limits bilaterally. Because of Mr. P.'s repetition difficulties, speech reception thresholds could not be tested. Instead, the Word Intelligibility by Picture Identification test (WIPI) (Ross & Lerman, 1971) was administered and showed excellent speech discrimination bilaterally (96 percent correct right ear, 92 percent correct left ear, at 50 dB HL).

SUMMARY OF SPEECH AND LANGUAGE FINDINGS

We found Mr. P. to have a severe verbal output disorder characterized by stuttering-like sound and syllable repetitions, some palilalia, and speech initiation problems accompanied by clonic-like spasms of the oral musculature. Conversational speech was often hypophonic and somewhat agrammatic. Few paraphasias were heard. Particular difficulties were noted on tests of auditory and reading comprehension, repetition, and writing. Confusion, set, and attentional problems also were prominent. He had mild limb and finger apraxia, but no buccofacial apraxia. Peripheral hearing was adequate for speech discrimination.

NEUROPSYCHOLOGICAL EVALUATION

A full neuropsychological evaluation showed that test performances were characterized by significant difficulty establishing, maintaining, and shifting set. According to the neuropsychology report, Mr. P. was impaired in most functions assessed, including "attention, mental control, response set, verbal and visuospatial intellectual functioning, visuospatial and constructional skills, and spatial memory." He earned a performance IQ of 79 on the Wechsler Adult Intelligence Scale—Revised (Wechsler, 1981). It should be noted that, despite these cognitive impairments, he was fully oriented to time and place and reportedly was able to perform all his activities of daily living. Verbal and functional memory were described as "operationally intact."

REEVALUATION ONE YEAR LATER

Upon completion of the initial evaluation, Mr. P. was discharged from the hospital, at his request, and returned to his job as a security guard. One year later, a speech and language evaluation showed the following changes. Spontaneous speech was noticeably more palilalic and dysfluent. Phrase length, as measured on the BDAE, had decreased from five words to three words, with concomitant reduction in grammatical form and melodic line. Production of automatic series was now limited to counting. Auditory comprehension was unchanged. It was Mrs. P.'s impression that her husband's speech and memory had deteriorated slightly, although he was still employed as a night security guard with apparently no social behavioral changes. Mr. P. reported that his headaches had increased in frequency and severity and that he was currently receiving chiropractic care.

DISCUSSION

Results from the speech–language and neuropsychological evaluations, in conjunction with Mr. P.'s history, neurological evaluation, and the CT scan information, suggested some form of progressive neurological illness of unclear etiology. Focusing on the prominent features of Mr. P.'s disorder, we considered several diagnoses.

Did Mr. P. have a stroke that resulted in "stammering speech," as questioned by the consulting physician?

As observed by the neurologist, Mr. P. displayed stuttering-like speech behavior. Neurogenic stuttering is associated with a variety of disorders, including multiple strokes, Parkinson's disease, tumor, closed head trauma, progressive supranuclear palsy, dementia, and drug use (Helm-Estabrooks, 1986). The stuttering, therefore, while symptomatic of a neurological problem, does not allow us to make a specific diagnosis in this case.

In addition, language testing showed a significant aphasia, with deficits in auditory comprehension, verbal expression, and repetition. Mr. P. had a history of hypertension and had experienced at least two brief episodes of speech arrest, which might suggest transient ischemic attacks (TIAs).

However, we ruled out a primary diagnosis of stroke given the history of progressive decline, the wide range of cognitive deficits found in neuropsychological testing, and the absence of a definitive focal lesion on the CT scan. This latter finding, along with the fact that there was not a "stair step" pattern of decline, led us to rule out multi-infarct dementia as well.

Could Mr. P. have progressive aphasia without generalized dementia?

Mesulam (1982) described a rare syndrome which he called "progressive aphasia without generalized dementia." The speech–language profile of patients with this syndrome includes slow, labored speech, frequent word-finding pauses, and usually an anomic aphasia. There are no accompanying deficits of intellect. Mr. P.'s speech was somewhat slow due to hesitations and stuttering, but he did not display the language characteristics of anomic aphasia. More important, he did have notable intellectual impairments. These facts rule out a diagnosis of progressive aphasia without generalized dementia. However, Wechsler (1977) described the case of a 67-year-old man with a degenerative dementia, whose first presenting symptom was a focal aphasic syndrome. Wechsler's impression was that the speech and language profile of this patient resembled the profile of a patient with classic fluent aphasia who produces paraphasias, neologisms, and jargon. Interestingly, a CT scan showed no focal lesion, but a strikingly dilated left sylvian fissure in the presence of moderate diffuse cortical atrophy. On the basis of the history and the CT findings, Wechsler diagnosed this patient as having either Pick's disease or Alzheimer's disease.

Does Mr. P. have Alzheimer's disease or Pick's disease?

As in Wechsler's case, Mr. P.'s first symptoms were in the speech-language sphere, and he showed evidence of significant dementia. Furthermore, his CT scan showed significant cortical atrophy. Did our patient have either of the two syndromes suggested by Wechsler, that is, Alzheimer's disease or Pick's disease? Certainly language problems are considered critical to the diagnosis of Alzheimer's disease and are commonly described in Pick's disease (Bayles & Kaszniak, 1987; Obler & Albert, 1981).

The severe naming impairment Mr. P. exhibited on the BNT and his impaired auditory comprehension are characteristic of Alzheimer's disease, but the striking dysfluency of his speech is not. Furthermore, recent memory, which is usually impaired even in early stages of Alzheimer's disease, was relatively preserved in Mr. P.

We then considered Pick's disease, a form of cerebral degeneration in which there is both cortical and subcortical atrophy (involvement). The speech and language characteristics of Pick's disease are relatively consistent with Mr. P.'s performance profile. Based on their review of the literature, Bayles and Kaszniak (1987) included the following speech and language characteristics in their description of Pick's disease:

- Slow, deliberate speech
- Dysnomia
- Defect in auditory comprehension
- Decrease in spontaneous output and mutism
- Breakdown of syntactic aspects of language
- Reading comprehension generally preserved
- Communication deficits more pronounced than memory deficits.

Similar characteristics were reported in Adams and Victor (1981):

> At first the patient speaks less but language is intact; later he or she may forget and misuse words and fail to understand much of what is heard or read. Speech becomes a "medley of disconnected words and phrases" and eventually is reduced to incomprehensible jargon. Finally the patient is altogether mute, seemingly without impulse or the ability to form words. Verbal perseveration, palilalia, and echolalia have been described. (p. 802)

Holland, McBurney, Moossy, and Reinmuth (1985) described the case of a man with Pick's disease whose speech was described as initially "stumbling" and paraphasic with frequent long pauses. He later progressed to mutism and gradually communicated only through writing. Auditory comprehension was reduced so that frequent repetition or careful attention to the speaker was required. Memory, cognitive functions, and social graces were relatively preserved until late in the course of the disease. Postmortem neuropathological evaluation revealed cortical atrophy, greater on the left than on the right, and particularly in the area of the left temporal lobe. Neurofibrillary tangles and Pick cells and bodies were seen. Adams and Victor (1981) also describe cortical and subcortical (i.e., "lobar") atrophy in Pick's disease, with atrophy of the frontal and temporal lobes most prominent.

Both Mr. P.'s speech–language findings and his CT scan are somewhat consistent with Pick's disease; that is, his impairment in auditory comprehension with frequent requests for repetition of questions and instructions, severe speech initiation problems, palilalia, and prominent frontal sulci and sylvian fissures. In addition, he displays the relative preservation of recent memory seen in Pick's disease. But to our knowledge, Mr. P. does not show any deterioration of work habits or social interactions commonly described as part of this syndrome (see Adams & Victor, 1981, for example). Holland's case, however, did not show social deterioration until many years into the disease.

The diagnosis of Pick's disease, then, appeared the best guess for our case. Still, given our patient's history and symptoms, we considered some rarer etiologies such as Parkinson-Dementia-ALS complex of Guam, and toxic metal encephalopathy.

Does Mr. P. have Parkinson-Dementia-ALS complex of Guam or toxic metal encephalopathy?

Based on Mr. P.'s history, two other rare disorders were considered. These were (1) the Parkinson-Dementia-ALS complex of Guam, because Mr. P. was stationed in Guam for one year, and (2) toxic metal encephalopathy, because Mr. P. was exposed to a number of metals in the tanning and paper industries. Indeed, some of Mr. P.'s findings are consistent with the Parkinson-Dementia-ALS complex of Guam; reduced initiation, visuospatial difficulties, and hypophonia. The striking dysfluency of Mr. P.'s speech, however, is not consistent with this disorder, nor does he show the bradykinesis or rigidity of this disease complex (Adams & Victor, 1981). Furthermore, this syndrome has not been described in non-natives who have briefly lived in Guam. Thus, this diagnosis seems highly unlikely.

More important, however, may be the 12 years Mr. P. spent in the tanning industry with exposure to aluminum salts and manganese. Some of the speech and language symptoms of aluminum intoxication (as, for example, in dialysis dementia) are hesitancy, stuttering dysarthria, aphasia, and sometimes apraxia of speech. Facial as well as generalized myoclonus may be present (Adams & Victor, 1981). Mr. P. presents with several of these symptoms— stuttering, aphasia, and facial dyskinesia (or myoclonus). Manganese poisoning can result in an extrapyramidal, post-encephalitic, Parkinson's-like syndrome with impassive facies, drooling, and monotonous, dysarthric speech (Adams & Victor, 1981). This picture however, is not consistent with Mr. P.'s present symptoms. In addition, a screening test for the presence of toxic metals was negative.

Several other rare disorders associated with progressive speech impairment were considered but ultimately ruled out. Among these were progressive supranuclear palsy, Whipple's disease, Huntington's disease, achromasia, general paresis, and Creutzfeldt-Jakob disease.

CONCLUSION

Although the etiology of Mr. P.'s disorder remains unknown, his case offered us the opportunity to test our differential diagnostic skills. In the end we decided that of the possible diagnoses, Mr. P.'s features were most consistent with Pick's disease, even though he failed to exhibit the characteristic personality and social behaviors of this disease. Follow-up evaluations over several years may lead to a more certain diagnosis, although Pick's disease is ultimately confirmed only by neuropathological examination of the brain.

Mr. P.'s case taught us the importance of several factors in the differential diagnostic process. Foremost among these factors were:

- The medical, vocational, and social history over the lifetime of the patient
- The team approach to examination of the patient, including neuroradiological, neuropsychological, and speech-language testing with final integration of all the evidence
- Access to, or familiarity with, literature pertaining to neurological disorders associated with speech and language changes.

REFERENCES

Adams, R.D., & Victor, M. (1981). *Principles of neurology* (2nd ed.). New York: McGraw-Hill.

Bayles, K.A., & Kaszniak, A.W. (1987). *Communication and cognition in normal aging and dementia.* San Diego: College-Hill Press.

Goodglass, H., & Kaplan, E. (1983). *The assessment of aphasia and related disorders* (2nd ed.). Philadelphia: Lea and Febiger.

Helm-Estabrooks, N. (1986). Diagnosis and management of neurogenic stuttering in adults. In K. St. Louis (Ed.), *The atypical stutterer.* Orlando, FL: Academic Press.

Holland, A.L., McBurney, D.H., Moossy, J., & Reinmuth, O.M. (1985). The dissolution of language in Pick's disease with neurofibrillary tangles: A case study. *Brain and Language, 24,* 36–58.

Kaplan, E., Goodglass, H., & Weintraub, S. (1983). *The Boston naming test.* Philadelphia: Lea and Febiger.

Mesulam, M-M. (1982). Slowly progressive aphasia without generalized dementia. *Annals of Neurology, 11,* 592–597.

Obler, L.K., & Albert, M.L. (1981). Language and aging: A neurobehavioral analysis. In D.S. Beasley & G.A. Davis (Eds.), *Aging: Communication processes and disorders.* New York: Grune & Stratton.

Ross, M., & Lerman, J. (1971). *Word intelligibility by picture identification (WIPI).* St. Louis: Auditec.

Wechsler, A.F. (1977). Presenile dementia presenting as aphasia. *Journal of Neurology, Neurosurgery, and Psychiatry, 40,* 303–305.

Wechsler, D. (1981). *Wechsler adult intelligence scale—revised.* New York: The Psychological Corporation.

Subject Index

Italic page numbers refer to tables and figures.

Notes

Notes

Notes

Notes

Notes

Notes